PR[A
SPILT MILK YOGA

"Reading this book, I felt I was with a warm, honest, and down-to-earth friend, sharing her insight and humor into what she aptly calls 'the volcanically active landscape' of family life. Cathryn Monro invites us to look deeply into our own experience and cultivate the qualities we most need as mothers to live our love—inner strength, flexibility, balance, and, most importantly, greater self-awareness."

—Myla Kabat-Zinn, coauthor of
Everyday Blessings: The Inner Work of Mindful Parenting

"A wise and insightful guide to embracing the transformative journey of motherhood as one of life's most profound gifts. *Spilt Milk Yoga* is the warm companion we need at our sides, connecting us to our own humanity as we navigate the constantly shifting terrain of tears, laughter, and learning. I wish someone had given this book to me when I was a new mum!"

—Shelley Davidow, author of *Raising Stress-Proof Kids*

"Cathryn Monro's passion for parenting and self-inquiry is woven into this practical and provocative tool for all mothers. Using recognizable, embarrassing, and often hilarious examples, *Spilt Milk Yoga* allows us to reveal our own truths, making us more open and ready to grow at the kitchen sink and beyond."

—Kate McIntyre Clere, director, *Yogawoman*

"I am a working mother of three, and Cathryn's inspirational book resonates with me on many levels. She achieves a universal message through the particular stories she tells. The ingenious workbook form provides a practical and clear pathway to deal with the issues mothers face, yet Cathryn's main concern is spirit and how we can light the way for ourselves and our kids."

—Miranda Harcourt, Order of New Zealand Merit, actor

"For readers who enjoy understanding life's transitions from a spiritual angle and are interested in a self-investigation into their mothering experiences, this book is a must."

—Laurie Hollman, PhD, psychoanalyst and author of
Unlocking Parental Intelligence

"I AM HOOKED! I so needed this—you have no idea! (Actually, you probably do!)

"I was having a trainwreck of a time as a mother, feeling unvalued and unseen and bad about my own mothering. I could never get it 'right.' *Spilt Milk Yoga* has helped me feel I am not alone, that there is a place to air the 'dark corners' of my experience, especially when I am struggling (which felt like always), and to know that I have my own wisdom. Reading *Spilt Milk Yoga*, I feel renewed determination and empowered to move forward. I am loving the motherhood journey in a completely new way.

"Straight to the point and no-nonsense, this book is super sustenance for me. It is simple and it goes in—even when I'm tired and stressed. I know my children benefit daily from this book as a resource for activating and remembering my inner wisdom. Reading *Spilt Milk Yoga*, I am learning that though it can be challenging and overwhelming at times, motherhood is the best mess there is, that there are small moments of joy if I take time to see them, that my life is not on hold until they 'grow up' and leave—my life is now.

Published by Familius LLC, www.familius.com

Familius books are available at special discounts, whether for bulk purchases for sales promotions or for family or corporate use. For more information, contact Premium Sales at 559-876-2170 or email orders@familius.com.

Library of Congress Cataloging-in-Publication Data
2016944195

Paperback ISBN 9781942934752
Ebook ISBN 9781944822194
Hardcover ISBN 9781944822200

Printed in the United States of America

Edited by Elena Gonzalez
Cover design by David Miles
Book design by Cathryn Monro, David Miles, and Brooke Jorden

10 9 8 7 6 5 4 3 2 1
First Edition

SPILT MILK
YOGA

FAMILIUS

To my mother, who has loved me with all her heart, and to my daughters, whom I love with all of mine.

SPILT MILK YOGA

A GUIDED SELF-INQUIRY TO FINDING YOUR OWN WISDOM, JOY, AND PURPOSE THROUGH

MOTHERHOOD

CATHRYN MONRO

CONTENTS

Chapters

To help you navigate *Spilt Milk Yoga: A Guided Self-Inquiry to Finding Your Own Wisdom, Joy, and Purpose through Motherhood* I've used the five *niyama*, the core actions of yoga, to organise the chapters. Translated as Self-Inquiry, Contentment, Self-discipline, Purity of Being, and Acknowledgement of the Spiritual Nature of Being. The *niyama* are interrelated and so are the chapters, so you'll find relevance and connections in whichever order you read them.

Part One—Swadhyaya: Self-Inquiry

Cultivating self-awareness, coming to know yourself honestly, inquiring as to why you do what you do, and reflecting on what moves you forward or holds you back.

Part Two—Santosha: Contentment

Cultivating acceptance of what is, of yourself and of others, being at peace with who you are right now, and finding contentment in any moment.

Part Three—Tapas: Self-Discipline

Cultivating your capacity to direct your energy purposefully, even when things get hot. The liberating fire of focus, intention, discipline, and perseverance.

Part Four—Shaucha: Purity of Being

Cultivating purity in mind, speech, and body. Decluttering your life and focusing on the good things that uplift and nurture your journey.

Part Five—Ishvarapranidhana: Acknowledging the Spiritual Nature of Being

Cultivating attitudes and behaviours that celebrate and uphold our appreciation of being. Being alive to the wonder of life; recognising that, in any small moment, we are part of something larger and that how we live is what makes our lives meaningful.

INTRODUCTION

Spilt Milk Yoga is the book I wish I'd had when I became a mother sixteen years ago. Being a mother has challenged and grown me in ways I never anticipated. It has been as hard and uncomfortable as it has been soft and loving. I have been pushed to the edges of my patience, anger, frustration, and purpose time and time again. At those times, a companion handbook linked to my questions, tears, and fears would've been more than welcome.

Spilt Milk Yoga draws on the principles and practices of yoga to shine light into the corners of motherhood we don't so easily talk about. The purpose of the book is connection—connection to self, to our own wisdom, joy, and purpose, to the value of motherhood as a site for engagement with our most profound development, as a path offering life's richest and most confronting lessons on love, acceptance, and joy.

Motherhood constantly confronts the edges of our self-knowing. We journey through an evolving and volcanically active landscape; violent, deep, and creative forces work in our subterranean selves. What stronger mirror of our habits and foibles, what better place to practise love, compassion, tolerance, and understanding than with ourselves and our children?

Yoga: *to yoke*. To yoke something is to harness its energy and turn it to good use. By consciously yoking the work we do as mothers to growing our self-knowledge, we align each to enrich the other. Together, they become the fuel and the lamp that illumines our path. Shine on!

How to Use *Spilt Milk Yoga*

Spilt Milk Yoga is written for you. If you have little children, cannot keep your tired eyes open at night, or are too busy getting through your day to read and process a whole book, just dip in and out. Open at the chapter that most speaks to your situation at the time and take what you need.

Each *Spilt Milk Yoga* chapter has four parts:

1. A quick grab quote
2. An account from my spilt-milk experience of mothering
3. A sustaining *Spilt Milk Yoga* practice to carry through your day
4. A page of guided self-inquiry for you to contemplate, respond to, develop, and record your practice (I recommend a 2B pencil for this job)

Spilt Milk Yoga is a companion to the conversation you have with yourself and foregrounds the importance of that conversation. Through the process of self-inquiry, naming concerns, asking questions of yourself, and contemplating your behaviours, assumptions, and choices, you develop understanding, purpose, and wisdom. When you appreciate the value and learning in your mothering journey, self-knowledge can unfold as you cook, clean, carry, cuddle, and curfew. The things you are wrestling with become the things you are awakening to: forgiveness, anger, judgement, maintaining inner peace.

Use *Spilt Milk Yoga* like a journal: write your self-inquiry responses in it, underline sentences that resonate, fold the corners of pages, add it to the nappy bag, and stick markers, notes from your kids, or images that uplift you in it. Having said that, use this book as it works for you. After all, it is your journey.

This Is NOT a Parenting Book

This is not a parenting book. There, I've said it twice. I'm no expert at parenting; I'm just doing my best and making a good enough job of it as you probably are too. There are many excellent parenting guides out there that give great advice about strategies for managing kids through bed-wetting, boundary-setting, chores, puberty, tantrums, sibling fights, pocket money, and much, much more.

But what do we do when the tantrum we're managing is our own? *Spilt Milk Yoga* looks at our journey as mothers and how we work with ourselves while we grapple with the challenges of motherhood. Motherhood drags us into the mire of our own shortcomings and offers us an opportunity to update old stories and catch negative habits. It offers countless opportunities to liberate ourselves as humans, to face those edges and grow wiser from the process of doing so. *Spilt Milk Yoga* is about capturing this wisdom to benefit us as we go.

Whether your child is two months old or fifteen years old, you are a mother on a unique journey with a job description that is broad and evolving. If we engage with it as a path to self-knowledge, motherhood can accelerate our learning and give us training as tough as any rigorous yoga master. We may not have time to sit at the feet of a teacher, but we are on a rich journey with our children and ourselves day to day. From it, we can learn what leads us toward living from a place of greater love, ease, tolerance, understanding, and joy.

Spilt Milk Yoga is a guide to tapping into and growing your own wisdom, which is in there, no matter how far away from it you may feel.

Why Spilt Milk?

Spilt milk happens. In motherhood, it happens in numerous ways; crayons on the wall, hoses in the window, cell phones "posted" into the toilet, five-year-old self-cut fringes on school photo day, litres of spectacularly spilt milk in aunty's new kitchen, through to shocking car accidents and painful disputes over baby names.

It's no use crying over spilt milk. The old adage suggests that what's done is done; get over it and get on with it. But if it's your milk that's spilt, and you've just spent two sleep-deprived hours slowly and painfully expressing it so you can leave your baby with her necessary feed while you attend to something else important, then crying may feel like the only available response. Or maybe the spilt milk is the indifferent mess left in the kitchen by your teen that, under the weight of household chores, sucker-punches your flare-up button.

There's the spilt milk, and then there's our response to it. The spilt milk is out of our control, but the response bit is up to us. That's the yogic part, our *sadhana*, our spiritual work. It's our choice how we respond; some responses hold us back, and some move us forward.

We could have wise and freeing responses to the spilt milk of our day. So why don't we? Our beliefs, histories, and proclivities shape our choices and behaviours, but they may not align with our longing for peace, joy, and connection. Investigating our internal world helps us move from how we reacted first off to what we'd like to do differently next time. If we engage purposefully with the many spilt milk events of our mothering days, we can practise more considered responses and be more alive to our choices next time. And there will be a next time. Spilt milk happens.

Why Yoga?

I've been a seeker of a better life all my life, for peace within, greater joy, liberation, and love. I was raised an atheist but with a deep appreciation for the miracle of being. Twenty-five years ago, I started practising yoga, just *asana*, poses, at first. Then I began to meditate, to engage in study and self-inquiry, and to read texts that would inspire and assist me to be a better person and to access more intention and happiness in my daily living.

Yoga encompasses conscious living on all levels—physical, emotional, psychological, spiritual, and environmental—through five *niyama*:

5. *Swadhyaya*: self-inquiry, reflection, self-education
6. *Santosha*: acceptance, satisfaction and contentment with what is, of yourself, and with others
7. *Tapas*: focus, intention, self-discipline, commitment
8. *Shaucha*: purity of being, inside and out, mind, speech, and body
9. *Ishvarapranidhana*: acknowledging the spiritual nature of being

These five actions and habits cultivate our well-being, enlightenment, and liberation. The pursuit of these actions through motherhood forms the basis of *Spilt Milk Yoga*. I'm not a certified yoga teacher or swami; I'm a mother, like you. I'm a fellow traveller, reaching out to share with you my hours of grappling and reflecting on the development of self-knowledge through motherhood. Motherhood, with all its rich and complex spilt milk, offers us a path to greater wisdom, joy, and purpose. Figuring out how and practising is the yoga.

My children reflect back instantly how I am being with them; if I am distracted, snappy, and unclear, the girls are "difficult." When I am open and positive, that's how I experience the world, and when I am anxious and contracted, that's how I experience the world.

The Five *Niyama* and ME!

I'm vacuuming. I'm feeling resentful that my fifteen-year-old is not doing something. I can't even remember what; it might've been homework, cleaning the bathroom, something. A battle of wills is going on. I can't even remember who started it. But I'm all wound up, so I'd put money on it having been me. Anyway, I'm right, of course! I'm feeling righteous and frustrated and unsupported, and I must've nagged or lectured or demanded. I sometimes do that; I march on in and accuse whoever of not helping me or doing what I want. I have a whole backstory simmering away on my inner stove, and then it's too much, the heat goes up just that bit more, I boil over, burst in, and spit out, "Can you at least clean the bathroom, or get off your chuff and DO SOMETHING!" Bang!

It's not a flattering habit, I know; actually, it's not really useful at all. Actually, it's more than not useful; it's destructive. This stewing and bursting is me splattering my frustration around as if the world should comply with my wishes, should succumb to my temper. I'm not taking care of the connections. My daughter pushes right back: "Mum, that is so rude! You should be modelling the behaviour that you want me to have."

How outrageous! How inflammatory! How antagonistic and rude and hypocritical and disrespectful and contrary and superior! And I am so shocked and furious at her behaviour. And I realise that it is my behaviour. And I know she's right. And I HATE being told this, having my awful behaviour thrown back at me by an uppity teenager. But I am sufficiently taken aback to swallow and say, "Thanks for pointing that out. Yup, that was awful. I'll try a different way next time." She is almost as gobsmacked as me.

The Five *Niyama* and YOU!

The five *niyama* are all to do with your relationship with yourself. As a mother, you will run up against yourself often. You'll be stretched, stressed, tired, frustrated, and challenged in some way that will call up your oldest and most base responses. Self-inquiry helps you catch yourself saying, doing, feeling, and thinking things that hinder your development, your freedom to live in the moment, and creates and opportunity to learn from them. **That's *swadhyaya*: self-inquiry, reflection, self-education.**

That's how it is; that's where you are. There is much to be appreciated in what you already have. **This is *santosha*: contentment, acceptance of what is, of yourself and of others.**

It's not a time to feel ashamed and crawl into a hole of self-hatred. It is a time to get to work, to embrace the chance to grow something new. What a great opportunity for an update, a more intentional approach, to practice doing things differently. **This is *tapas*: the fire of focus, intention, discipline, and perseverance.**

Once you've turned your attention to your habits, you can choose to cultivate new ones that support and uplift your journey. **This is *shaucha*: purity of being in mind, speech, and body.**

Of course, this will have an effect on much more than you; it will affect your experience of the world and of your children, and the experience your children have of you. You are your own closest companion, with yourself at every moment; through yourself, you experience this miracle of being. **This is *Ishvarapranidhana*: acknowledging and celebrating the spiritual nature of being.**

The Five *Niyama*: Inquiry

Note down below how practising each of the five *niyama* could benefit your life as a mother this week. Consider what you could do for each one, what you might have to give up, and what you might gain.

Swadhyaya: self-inquiry, reflection, self-education

Santosha: contentment, acceptance of what is, of yourself and of others

Tapas: focus, intention, discipline, and commitment

Shaucha: purity of being in mind, speech, and body

Ishvarapranidhana: acknowledging and celebrating the spiritual nature of being

PART ONE

Swadhyaya

SELF-INQUIRY

WHAT AM I DOING, AND WHY?

When I shine light into my dark corners, I find nothing stronger there than me.

SPILT MILK

I HAT MUM is gouged in red pen capitals on a purple post-it note and mashed onto my bedroom door. It's a clear message. My youngest is unhappy with my mothering decision to set a boundary and say "no" to a playdate. A bit of hate mail for doing what I think is right isn't going to bring my world down, especially with that rather endearing spelling mistake. I know what this is about. I can take this. I feel clear, steady, understanding of her response.

But sometimes the notes I send myself about my mothering are not amusing, endearing, or reasonable in their context. I'm standing, panicking, in a blizzard of toys and breakfast dishes. *What a mess! Get your act together* comes the message. I'm hanging out a wash or clearing a half-eaten dinner; tired, I want to stop. *You've done nothing worthwhile all day* says the note. I'm sitting on an icepack breastfeeding my newborn with swollen, aching breasts, feigning interest in my three-year-old's cartwheel show. *If my master's degree supervisor could see me now . . .* I imagine him shaking his head disparagingly: "Is this all you amounted to?" I am caught between forcing my distraught ten-year-old out of the car to play soccer to not let the team down, or listening to her wailing distress about not having brushed her hair and being too tired to play after a late night sleepover. *I should know what to do and do it!* comes the pressured admonishment. I feel judged. I judge myself. I feel shaken, doubtful, undermined.

What I really want in those moments is internal support, to appreciate what I am doing, to embrace the not knowing lightheartedly, to have my judgement guide me toward living more freely and lovingly.

Self-Inquiry

Samskara saksat karanat purvajati jnanam.
Through sustained focus and meditation on our patterns, habits, and conditioning, we gain knowledge and understanding of our past and of how we can change the patterns that aren't serving us, to live more freely and fully.
—Patanjali, Yoga Sutra III.18

❝ . . . to live more freely and fully." Doesn't that sound great! This ancient verse tells you how to do it, too: "through sustained focus and meditation on our patterns, habits, and conditioning."

The essential practice of *Spilt Milk Yoga* is self-inquiry. Through self-inquiry, you gain knowledge about what you do and why. Sustained inquiry develops awareness of your habits, frees up new options, and reinforces fresh understanding.

The feelings and thoughts you have about yourself as a mother are yours, and you have to work and live with them every day. Where do they come from? What messages about mothering do they send you? Are they working for you?

Asking yourself questions and attempting to answer them will focus your awareness and shine light into the corners of beliefs so deep within your view of the world that they are hard to recognise. Self-inquiry makes space for you to think and feel things through. No one else will be checking your work, but you will.

At the end of the day, you have to live with yourself—and wouldn't you rather it be a loving, honest, and supportive relationship?

SELF INQUIRY: INQUIRY

Write down three attributes you want to develop in yourself through being a mother.

Write down three messages you send yourself that assist you developing these.

Write down three messages you send yourself that get in the way of you developing these.

When you reflect on the things you've written above, what do you notice about even this small piece of self-inquiry?

What is one thing from this inquiry you could carry into your mothering day to help you live more freely and fully?

Great. So that's the start!

2

WILL MOTHERHOOD RUIN MY LIFE?

Inner work involves a lot of self-effort: asking hard questions, examining intentions and actions, and working to give up restrictive behaviours. A spiritual life supports you in living a life of love, connection, and joy.

SPILT MILK

I was raised with a good dose of feminism. I wanted to do something worthwhile with my life. I had a picture of myself as an independent, professional, self-directed career woman, capable and educated. I also had a picture of myself as a mother.

I am six years old playing in a neighbour's playhouse, playdough in the frying pan on the wooden stove, my dolly wrapped in a hanky in a wooden rocking cradle nearby. I am playing the role of mother: busy, purposeful, and content.

I am sixteen, aware of life being more complex. Life is about choices, autonomy, education, and cutting my own path. What career will make me feel purposeful and content? How am I going to put playdough on the table? I am horrified at a school friend having a baby and not going to university. I don't want to "waste my life." (Can you spot the upcoming predicament?)

I am thirty-six. My conflicting beliefs about the value of mothering have left me holding the baby and the bathwater. I am supposed to be a cracking career woman and an attentive, engaged, present mother, but it is not possible to do both concurrently to the level I expect of myself. My socio-political values are not connected with my socio-biology. Hello spilt milk, hello tears.

I am forty, scanning the indexes of books by swamis, monks, and spiritual teachers for references to motherhood, parenting, children, family—anything that will illuminate and give value to the Sisyphean tasks of my daily mothering life. Then it dawns on me that none of these teachers are mothers. So how can I translate these teachings and with them embrace the particular challenges I meet in my journey through motherhood?

Check Your Inner Approach

Your inner journey is supremely valuable in living the life you want. Motherhood is an epic inner journey, requiring service and sacrifice as you face myriad demons of frustration, rage, guilt, exhaustion, and intolerance, all the while carrying other beings who depend on you to get through. Motherhood is not easy, but it is very important.

Yoga means a forcible joining together of two things. Once you have a child, you are a mother; there is no going back. You are joined to the work of mothering. How you turn to that work and its demands is defined by your ideas, beliefs, and attitude to mothering. Are the early years an endurance test of boredom and drudgery or a chance to feel what it is like to be the life-giver, protector, primary companion, and most-important-person-in-the-world to an unfolding soul? Is motherhood a frustrating hiatus in your career while you itch to get back to work or a chance to experience the ageless rhythm of life beyond the confines of the trade and industry paradigm? Are the teenage years filled with regret that you didn't appreciate the earlier ones, or the adventure of being alongside while your blossoming young adult navigates the world, secure in the knowledge of your steadfast love?

The practice here is check your inner approach. If you are seeking fulfilment of some deeper personal purpose—happiness, ease, lightness, presence—you can engage with motherhood as a path to attaining it, to living the life you want not *after* motherhood but *because* of it. Motherhood is a rich source of reflection on your habits, patterns, and conditioning and an opportunity to grow your most realised self. Your inner approach to motherhood can fuel your journey to self-realisation and contribute to the fulfilment of your highest human potential.

CHECK YOUR INNER
APPROACH: INQUIRY

Describe your current life as a mother and how you feel about it.

What hopes and expectations do you have for your life as a mother?

What questions do you have about your current life as a mother?

Take one of these questions. What is your inner approach to this question; what do you think and feel about it?

What beliefs about your inner journey support you as a mother?

What beliefs about motherhood support you in your inner journey?

Review your question above. Note any shifts in your inner approach toward it and what inner approach you want to carry into your day.

3

THE SHOCK OF BIRTH

*While you love and raise
your child, you can raise your
tolerance for your own humanity
and divinity.*

SPILT MILK

iving birth was a shock. I'd read about it; I'd heard about it; I'd even assisted a friend giving birth. She had shouted in my face point-blank, "NO ONE EVER TOLD ME IT WAS GOING TO BE LIKE THIS!" I heard that loud and clear, and I got prepared. But as much as I'd primed myself with antenatal classes, yoga, advice from others, and a birth plan, nothing prepared me for the psychic shock of it. Despite glimpsing its shadowy presence on an ultrasound scan and the growing discomfort and inconvenience of hosting its expanding tenancy, my baby was still somewhat of a concept until I saw her head emerging in the midwife's wavering mirror. I had *imagined* what it would be like to be a mother. I had pictured snapshots of the life ahead of me. But I was still shocked. Nothing could really have prepared me for it.

I was shocked that a complete person came out of my body, so finished and separate. I'm not sure what I expected, but her entirety blew me away. Her own lungs, ears, fingernails, all working. Then it hit me that now I had to care for this vulnerable being. It was all up to me, and I didn't know what to do. The responsibility I felt to my baby eclipsed all else. I was in complete service to the survival of this mystifying, tiny person. I understood my biology in a new way; it overrode rational thought and shattered my previously independent self. From the first moment she was laid on my chest, a new Me was also born, Me as mother, the responsible half of an intertwined lifelong duo, no longer autonomous and separate. My whole life flipped. I scrambled to reconfigure my life around another person. It consumed me moment to moment, day to day. Things that used to matter didn't matter anymore. I forgot my birthday. Lost and found, there was a deeply met part of me too. To this day, watching my children eat broccoli satisfies me as much as if I'd eaten it myself.

Embracing the Learning

Becoming a mother is a huge transition, and it can be a struggle to adapt. Your body changes, your focus and lifestyle change, your priorities and worries change, and your identity changes. Change is truly the only constant. As your child develops and changes rapidly, you will constantly be in uncharted territory, making it up as you go along, looking for the answer only to find the question has changed.

The practice here is embracing the learning. Embracing the learning acknowledges that you are on a journey; you cannot know everything in advance, but the learning is coming. Having a learner's mind is at the heart of this first *niyama* of self-inquiry. To cultivate self-knowledge requires learning, and honest inquiry into your own experience can be revealing and unsettling.

It is not widely shared that becoming a mother can be shocking, difficult, and frightening. The surprise of it can be disorienting. You may feel you are losing your mind or drowning in expectations you cannot meet. Amongst it all, know that motherhood is a fast track to self-knowledge; it will shower you in opportunities to go with the flow even as you spin in an eddy of doubt and confusion. Know that you have what it takes to be a mother. When you embrace the learning in front of you, you will find that motherhood is a powerful force for growing you up in a whole new way. You are encountering another aspect of life's incredible richness, entering a territory where love and fear learn to shake hands, listen to each other, and converse wisely. As a student of life, things just got way more interesting!

EMBRACING THE LEARNING: INQUIRY

Describe the impact on you of becoming a mother. How did your life change?

What have you developed as a result of this?

What are you currently finding challenging in your life as a mother?

What might the learning be from this?

What are you appreciating about your life as a mother?

What is one small thing you could do in your day to honour this?

4

I'M A MOTHER!
WHAT DO I DO NOW?

*Did you meet that new situation
adequately or that old situation with
something new? That is enough.
That is the best you can do.*

SPILT MILK

I t is my first day home alone with my new baby. I watch my husband drive off to work in our little yellow Datsun. Away, down the road, and around the corner. Gone. A panicky void opens in my gut. What am I supposed to do now? I don't know what to do.

I'm a mother. I have a baby. But it doesn't mean I know what to do. Everyone acts as if it's so natural, as if I should automatically know how to swaddle, what a tired sign looks like, when to feed her, when to put her down, what "normal" crying is. But I don't. I don't even know about tired signs yet. There is no manual. There is just me and my baby. It is all completely new. I am at sea.

I walk back inside, every step resounding in my skull. It feels like conducting slow-motion, open-heart surgery, like someone's life depends on me, which it does, but I'm untrained. It's guesswork.

I get through my day adequately. Check sleeping baby. *Is she okay?* Wash nappies. Check sleeping baby. *Does she need to wake soon for a feed? I don't know.* Check email. She wakes. Breastfeed her. *Enough? I don't know.* Hold her. Marvel at her being, her ears, her smell. Talk to and nuzzle her. I can do that bit. But I'm winging the logistics. *Check and change her nappy? Put her back to bed?*

Fifteen years later, I look back and think how much I learned, how now I'd have more of an idea of what to do. And yet I'm still faced with newness. My fifteen-year-old asks to go to a New Year's party with a friend; there will be alcohol and people I don't know. I'm at sea again. There is no manual . . .

Collaborating with Life

You cannot prepare in advance for all motherhood will throw at you. You will meet the old and the new, your knowing and not-knowing, and have plenty of opportunities to train on the job in responding to the moment. This is life, unfolding as it will.

The practice here is collaborating with life, meeting life with the spontaneity and creativity with which it created you. Spontaneity is the creative and life-affirming act of doing something new in an old situation or something adequate in a new situation. Did you ever react and think *I could have done that better* then relived that situation in your mind, figuring what you could've said, imagining yourself responding differently? This is you creating options for yourself to collaborate more readily with life next time.

Through self-inquiry, you come to understand which responses free you and which ones restrict you. It is enough to respond to a new situation adequately, without fragmenting. It is enough to respond to an old situation in a new way, affirming life's inherent creativity in the face of restriction. Increasing your options gives you freedom to respond in alignment with your values and conscious intentions rather than out of old reactive unconscious habits. Collaborating with life requires that you appreciate the creativity of your responses in any moment. Ask yourself, *Did I do something new in an old situation, or something adequate in a new situation?* If the answer is *yes*, rejoice in your creativity. If the answer is *no*, feel yourself waking up to the possibilities life is offering you. There is no right or wrong response to this collaboration, only your next offer, and your next, and your next . . .

COLLABORATING WITH LIFE: INQUIRY

Consider a current or recent mothering experience where you were faced with a new situation. What about it was new?

What was your response?

Was your response adequate? In what way?

Consider a current or recent mothering moment where you were faced with an old situation. What was your response?

Was your response new? In what way?

Take one of these moments. What could you appreciate about what you are creating in collaboration with life?

What can you carry forward into your day from this inquiry?

5

HOW DO I GET THERE FROM HERE?

*With intention as your compass,
you will always be travelling in
the right direction.*

SPILT MILK

I'm in the back garden. It's a nice day. My six-year-old is jumping on the trampoline. My three-year-old, who is a little less predictable in her ricochet trajectories, gets on too. It is a delightful, playful, good thing to do. It's also tinged with danger, anxiety, and a high possibility of things going wrong. I am enforcing turn-taking. I am keeping them safe. I am on hand to catch, guide, observe, encourage, rescue, represent in the negotiations, educate in good citizenship and loving relationships. Play is complex work!

I am also thinking that it'd be good to hang out the washing, that I need to get ready for the next thing, that I need a shower and to shop for dinner, and that, deep down, I want a break. I'd like to be hanging with another adult, perhaps at a workplace, or in my studio, doing my thing. I can't let go of the feeling that I want to be somewhere else. Yup, I'm frustrated, stuck, feeling my potential going to waste.

Of course, being with my children is wonderful—mostly, in fact. Wonderment and joy are a big part of our days together. I don't want them to ever think I resented mothering them or felt burdened by them. It is my own thoughts and habits burdening me. I want to be with my children and clear of the burden. I know there is no substitute for being here, putting my all into this important work of play. But in this moment, I don't feel fulfilled, stilled, at peace. I feel life is passing me by, happening somewhere else. I feel torn, underutilised.

Is this the thing: that fulfilment is in any moment regardless of place and task? I imagined the prerequisites for fulfilment to be so much grander than this. It is good, this moment, but I am unclear about my purpose.

Intention

Intention, conscious or not, is behind every action. Becoming aware of your intention can lift you out of the rut of an old habit onto a more enlightened path. A conscious intention is like a compass that orients you to your true north. In new situations, intention will guide you where you have no map. Without conscious intention, you are more likely to react to pressure in the moment, to make haphazard and inconsistent decisions, and to feel doubtful that you are going in the right direction.

The practice here is intention. Being intentional means you are more able to choose the actions that shape your life. To form intention, it is necessary to tune into what you are wanting to develop, what you aspire to, and the goals you may have in any situation. It is important to frame it in the positive. Rather than something you are trying NOT to do (*To not compare myself to others*), make it something to DO (*To stay centred in my own worth*). From here, you have something to hold onto in challenging moments.

To appreciate the joy and worth of this moment of play.
To stay steady in the face of my child's anger.
To be present when my child comes to me for a cuddle.
To value the good things I provide for my child.

The vaguer your intention, the vaguer the result. The more purposeful your intention, the more purposeful the result. Having a clear intention enables clearer choices in any moment, a sense of growth when you're on the right track to your goal. Your intention will change and develop, but the practice is to be conscious of your intentions nonetheless.

INTENTION: INQUIRY

Write down a recent mothering situation you found challenging. What was challenging about it for you?

What are you wanting to develop in moments like this?

Turn this into a statement of intention. (Remember to frame it in the positive.) My intention is to:

Put the above two answers into a statement.
In my life as a mother, I am practising:

So that:

What is one way you could you practise this intention in your mothering day today?

6

MOTHERHOOD AND A SPIRITUAL LIFE?

As a mother, your life is rich in opportunities for spiritual growth. Motherhood will hold you to commitment like nothing else will, hold you to tolerance, patience, thoughtfulness, consideration, compassion, self-inquiry, self-restraint, and love.

SPILT MILK

I used to be able to sit and meditate in peace. Okay, even if I didn't get around to it, at least I had the option. *My home is my ashram*, I say to myself, but there's nothing divine about bath time at my house tonight, the tussle over the puppy soft toy, competing bedtime story needs, a benchful of dishes, and my own yearning for a sense of achievement. I long for calm, but I'm lost in a maze of chores and immediate needs. HOW and WHERE and WHEN do I fit in my spiritual life? Have my inner-yogi-seeker and I parted ways?

I picture my unlived life walking resolutely up the pathway. I'm a soul on a quest for spiritual enlightenment with nothing but a longing for liberation from petty concerns. Foregoing material comforts and family relationships, I exchange silks for loincloth and begging bowl. I pilgrimage to a sacred river, teacher, or mountain. Leading a life of austerity and discipline, I engage in tests of mind over matter, endure blistering sun and freezing wind, naked, fasting and meditating until I pass into transcendence. But I'm a contemporary Western woman and that's not my life, as I cut up fruit and set out water-play. Or what about: cloistered in a quiet chapel, I forgo secular marriage and motherhood and, freed from this common social script, live my days quietly gardening, serenely contemplating my spiritual being? Well, obviously, that's not me either, as my toddler wakes and cries and her short afternoon sleep scuppers plans to have an hour inhabiting my atrophying professional identity.

So what is my spiritual life? It's certainly not a life of seclusion, hours of quiet meditation, or whispered conversations in the porticoes! There is no time to sit, and peace is hard to imagine. I'm lucky to finish a sentence without interruption, a cup of tea before it is cold, or a page of my own choice. Surely there's just as much grist for my spiritual mill in the ordinary, testing, selfless, real, and insightful journey of my mothering days? But how do I grasp it?

Working with What You've Got

I n yoga, it is widely held that we all have it within us to progress. Amongst saints and seekers of many traditions are all sorts of ordinary people: a householder, a barber, a baker, a prostitute. There are many ways to live a spiritual life. You do not have to leave behind your life to find your path. You are already on it. What makes a life spiritual? How you approach it.

Motherhood is as worthy a spiritual life as any other and provides plenty of opportunities for endurance, restraint, discipline, and sacrifice; it is a teacher of patience, a mountain of mirroring, an endurance test of selflessness, a cleansing river of love. Every day is ripe with challenges to see beyond the mundane dramas of the world and engage with greater meaning and purpose.

The practice here is working with what you've got. Engage with your experiences of motherhood as nutrients for your spiritual garden. Gather up all those doubts and blunders as rich compost to sustain and nourish your spiritual journey. Every mothering mess-up is valuable if you learn from it!

Motherhood can be as valuable a path as any other, depending on your approach. Upholding motherhood as a spiritual journey makes your contribution to the world a daily one. You can reduce suffering and increase joy right here and now within your world, right in amongst the many spilt milk moments of your mothering life.

WORKING WITH WHAT YOU'VE GOT: INQUIRY

What are you seeking in life?

How does being a mother contribute to this?

Recall a recent mothering moment where you felt challenged in the areas you are seeking. How did you respond?

What did you learn in this situation?

What is one thing you will do in your day today to recognise the spiritual value of your journey as a mother?

7

DON'T INTERRUPT ME;
I'M TRYING TO BE
SPIRITUAL

*Stay alive to your potential in
this moment, commit to being
aware of what is in front of you,
and listen with your subtle ears
to the wisdom inside you.*

SPILT MILK

pace to myself is rare. No sooner than I sit to meditate, work, chant, contemplate, or go to the loo, I'm interrupted. I prep my kids and tell them I'm taking a minute to myself and finally sit down to listen to a lesson on contemplation. The theme is "seeing God in each other." I've just settled in when my daughter comes in asking me to get her some water. I am annoyed and irritated. *Can't she see that what I'm doing is important? What about me? Can't she get the glass of water herself?*

Fortunately, I'm a little more open to insight than I was before I sat down, so I don't just react. I take a deep breath and manage to grasp that perhaps this moment is food for contemplation. Squinting through a lens of acceptance, love, and tolerance, I can see this interruption instead as an offering. Her coming in now becomes part of this lesson: seeing God in each other. Here she is. God is in her. Asking for a glass of water.

What this person is asking of me is what God is asking of me. What I tell this person is what I tell God. How I respond to this person is how I respond to God. I could ask her lovingly to wait, and I can even appreciate the interruption as an opportunity to practise seeing God in another person, to see my daughter in her divinity.

I get up and get her some water. But instead of being angry, resentful, or unkind, I feel light. I am happy to do it. It is a sweet moment. Here is God in this lovely little person. I feel the benefit of the contemplation even if it was only two minutes long, and perhaps more so because it was interrupted. The deepest wonderment of life's expression is right in front of me as my daughter.

Contemplation—Accessing the Wisdom inside You

Motherhood is full of questions and concerns big and small. Often, the questions are complex and the answers not one size fits all. Wisdom is easier to access from a place of steady thoughtfulness rather than a state of pressured anxiety or frustration.

The practice here is contemplation. Contemplation is an act of tapping into your own wisdom. Contemplation is a process of trusting in the creativity of life. Contemplation turns a concern into a question, a problem into something you can work with. When you respond steadily to your anxious mind, you make space for wisdom to arise.

To contemplate, identify something your mind is chewing on: *I am worried about my child's unhappiness at school.* Turn your concern into a question: *How do I best support my child out in the world?* It can be a very specific practical or personal question: *Shall I take on this part-time work? How should I approach this person? What does my anger about this event tell me?*

Take a moment to sit quietly. Hold your question in your mind, and when you have it in your steady focus, let it hover. In the space that opens around your question, allow for the creativity of your wisdom. Don't be in a rush. If you get interrupted, know that you have begun the process. Wait and see what emerges. Let things come. Notice any judgements: *Oh, that was too quick, too easy an answer; this isn't working; what if nothing comes . . .?* and just hold the space of contemplation open and listen gently. Your inner wisdom may surface straight away, it may take a few days, it may be faint or strong, or it may be another question. Wisdom is in you; listen for it.

CONTEMPLATION—ACCESSING
THE WISDOM INSIDE YOU:
INQUIRY

Write down any current concerns and questions you have for contemplation.

Take one and turn it into a question for contemplation.

Write down what you know about this question, situation, or concern.

Take a few minutes to sit comfortably and close your eyes. Hold the question in your mind, offering it up for a response. Listen gently. Write down what emerges.

If you don't have time to sit and quiet is not available right now, simply form a question and let it go. Come back in two days or a week and note what has emerged since.

8

MAKING MISTAKES: I'M TRYING TO DO RIGHT, BUT I'VE DONE IT WRONG

Compassion is kind-heartedness and care. What greater approach can you have on this journey? While you practise and learn, compassion will carry you forward.

SPILT MILK

You might cut your baby's skin when you first cut her fingernails. I did. You may accidentally get sunblock in her eyes. I did. You may even have, just yesterday, exploded in frustration and, in order to drive home a healthy food–choice point, done a very bad, high, left-handed slam-dunk with a packet of offending chocolate biscuits, meant to get the bin, but missed and hit the bench, resulting in smashed biscuits, a startled fourteen-year-old, a bemused husband, an ashamed mother . . . yup, I did. Not one of my better mothering moments.

I'm trying to do right. But I've done it wrong.

Reason: I'm furious at my daughter snacking on chocolate biscuits at breakfast time. Why: because I put so much effort into educating my kids about good and bad choices so that they will have gloriously healthy lives. Underneath: I had compromised at the supermarket and bought a lunchbox treat. Underneath that: I feel my generosity is not appreciated. Under that: I feel hurt and angry at myself that I gave in. My belief: informed food choice is important. The moment: a dramatic display of the depth of my conviction and a demand to be listened to and respected, dammit! Effect: broken biscuits, damaged reputation as expert on anger management, poor role-modelling. But? Perhaps at least eating chocolate biscuit lunchbox treats for breakfast is now on the agenda as NOT OKAY!

That was my aim, but now it's tangled in my outburst of frustration, my shame at my own behavior, and my sense of being unappreciated. Will the ends justify the means?

Compassionate Learning

Motherhood requires learning on the job. Learning happens when you come to the edge of what you know. Not knowing what to do has its own dance of pressure, expectation, and doubt.

You will make mistakes as a mother. Making mistakes is part of learning. You will encounter many challenges and much learning around managing your child's sleep, feeding, childcare, birthday parties, homework, course choices, lunchboxes, school, friends, screen time. Just when you've learned about bedtime for a three-month-old, they turn four months or six or fifteen years old and the goalposts move. Then there is managing your own sleep, friends, boundaries, self-worth, sense of doing it right or wrong, need for appreciation. There will be times you don't know how and what to do because you haven't been in this situation before, and if an issue seems to be repeating, well, there's more to learn.

The practice here is compassionate learning. Accept and value making mistakes as part of your progress and learning. Learning is challenging: you try something; it may work well, it may not. When you make a mistake, try feeling compassion for yourself rather than shame; try appreciation of your efforts and learning over harsh judgement. You are doing your best. Suspend or befriend judgement and focus instead on what you are practising and learning.

Compassion reduces pressure and acknowledges learning as the practice that will carry you forward. You are learning; mistakes are invaluable teachers. Treat yourself and your learning with care and compassion.

COMPASSIONATE LEARNING:
INQUIRY

Recall a recent mothering moment when you didn't know what to do, made a mistake, or got something "wrong." What happened, and how did you respond?

What are you learning from this mothering situation?

What are you wanting to move from? What are you wanting to move toward?

If you practise having compassion for yourself, what changes?

With **compassionate learning**, what might you do differently next time?

What from this inquiry can you carry into your day today?

9

OVERLOAD

How do you want to be with this precious breath; how do you want to be in this precious moment, right here and now?

SPILT MILK

I am chopping vegetables, frying onions, putting on a load of washing, doing the dishes, taking a phone call about setting up tomorrow morning's Playcentre session, pushing baby in a swing hung in the kitchen doorway, watching my four-year-old's fairy ballerina dance, and running the bath all at the same time. With that much going on, it takes very little to upend a bag of frozen peas, knock over a glass of milk, and flood the bathroom. The spilt milk adds to the list of things to attend to NOW, and to my stress. I'm sweeping up peas, mopping up spilt milk . . . OMG THE BATH!!!

I'm living in a state of inner franticness, trying to do it all really well. Even if I stop and watch my fairy ballerina and attempt to give her the attention she wants, or turn off the bath or washing machine, the tasks don't go away; the washing just sits there, and the dinner still needs to be cooked. I feel if I stop swimming, I'll go under. I don't know how to stop; there is so much I have to do.

I have a clear hour but find myself still rushing and spinning in circles with *what to do next?* Should I check emails, vacuum, fold, put away the washing? I find it almost impossible to shake the sense of rushing and just relax.

I'm in overload, just holding on. I'm chanting the stress mantra *C'mon. C'mon. C'mon.* as I herd the kids from one place to another, anxiously pre-planning my next step. I'm clenching my teeth at night. My dentist asks, "Do you have a stressful job?" I feel fraudulent, pathetic, angry. I know I'm not CEO of globalimportance.com, but actually, yes, I do. I am a mother, and I'm finding it a stressful job. I don't know how else to do it.

Assessing What Matters

Y ou will have many demands on your time, many responsibilities, and many tasks as a mother. And you will take them seriously because they matter to you. Caring for your children, dishes, laundry, reading stories, cooking, feeding, shopping, making beds, and much, much more are the essential and unavoidable tasks of mothering. You may have help with these, or not; you may have different tasks, additional tasks, sick parents, paid work, or other things that add to your load.

A wise monk said, "An overloaded boat is easily capsized by wind and waves." If you are feeling overloaded, it is important that you listen to this feeling. Allow for the reality of the essential load you already carry, and consider what you could do to lighten your load. Loading up your boat with extra tasks and expectations may weigh you down unnecessarily and compromise your balance and buoyancy in the wind and waves of your mothering day. It may be practical things adding to your load—the gymnastics class across town that your child complains about every Tuesday—or an inflexible or uncompromising idea—*I HAVE to provide a nutritious home-cooked meal every day for my children; I SHOULD be able to cope with this*—or perhaps it is a habit that creates more load on your day: doing one-more-thing before you get out the door, saying "yes" to unpaid jobs where "no" might have be the better answer, or trying to do too much between five and seven p.m.

The practice here is assessing what matters. If overloaded is not how you want to live, examine your load. Is there anything in your load that you could do without? Travelling more lightly through your day will enable you to enjoy being a mother more, to prioritise your joy, to love and value what really matters to you.

ASSESSING WHAT MATTERS: INQUIRY

Write out a list of what you have to do today. Then go through and mark each thing (A) absolutely essential, (B) semi-important, or (C) not important.

Note next to each thing when you expect to do it. What do you notice about the shape of your day?

Now add in anything else that adds to your load: expectations, habits, ideas.

Describe what overload is like for you.

Instead of overload, what do you choose for yourself today?

What could you do to lighten your load today?

Try it. At the end of the day, note here what you learn and what you'd like to try next.

PART TWO

Santosha

CONTENTMENT

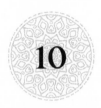

10

RUSHING, GETTING
NOWHERE FAST

*The still point in your
day can be you!*

SPILT MILK

My kids are driving me crazy with their whining; I am stressed about all I have to do before I do the things I really have to do. I can't conceive of how to fit even five minutes' meditation into my frantic day. Every minute has multiple claims on it from a multitude of directions: the immediate and unavoidable demands of mothering, parenting, housework, administration, career . . . each section has its own endless list. I feel overwhelmed minute by minute and stretched in different directions. Even if my day is only busy and not frantic, five minutes to myself seems impossible. In which moment do I focus? Where do I focus? What do I pay attention to? My day is a blur of events. I am rushing to keep up.

I cannot focus on one thing because so many things are happening in any moment. I am simultaneously with the lost hairbrush event, the waking-my-child-up-to-responsibility-for-her-own-hairbrush event, the burnt toast event, the event breaking out over the last bagel, the unkind word event, the clock ticking toward EXIT o'clock . . . I am supervisorally responsible for it all: food choice, late homework, shoes that fit, nails cut, talks about friendship, about pet death, about sex, for constructive feedback and exploding sensitivity, the big and small of it all, the short and long term of it all. All of it is important.

And if I make myself sit down amidst it all, I'm so agitated that "sitting for meditation" is another "thing to do." I do not feel calm when I sit. My heart is thumping. I feel frustrated, panicky. I could be DOING something on my TO-DO lists, like hanging out the wash. A sense of pressure pervades my mind. My body is tense. Sitting still is the last thing I feel like doing.

Slowing Down

L onging for inner calm? If your day feels chaotic, you will need a still point to come back to. It is hard to respond steadily when you are off-centre. Like an unbalanced washing machine clunking out in the spin cycle, you need to stop, rearrange your load, and get balanced so you can continue, more able to do your job as a mother from the calm, still point of your centre. To find your centre in the rush, you have to slow down.

The practice here is slowing down. If you are tussling with where to put your focus or overwhelmed in the jumble of your day, then slowing down your inner speed will create more space for appreciation, awareness, and acceptance. From a place of inner steadiness, you are more likely to get things done effectively.

Sit if you can, but if you can't, just start with mindful breathing. Take three slow deep breaths all the way in, all the way out. Notice how you are feeling and simply name the feelings as they arise and subside:

This feeling is resistance. This feeling is irritation. This feeling is overwhelm. This feeling is happiness. This feeling is exhaustion. This feeling is self-pity. This feeling is guilt. This feeling is despair. This feeling is relief.

You may cook resentfully or contentedly, you may sit to meditate angrily or joyfully, but rather than thinking *I'll rush through this, then I'll slow down,* turn your mind to the quality of your being while you carry out the task. In connecting to the self through which your feelings ebb and flow, you will have to slow down. Rather than focusing on the chore or fighting yourself, simply recognise your state, connect to the self that observes, and watch what happens inside you.

SLOWING DOWN: INQUIRY

Practise slowing yourself down now using the breath. Take three deep breaths all the way in and all the way out. Relax your jaw, your shoulders; let go of all that and breathe naturally. Note briefly what arises in you.

Take a few moments to recognise and name your feeling state.
This feeling is . . .
This feeling is . . .
This feeling is . . .
This feeling is . . .

What effect does naming your feelings have on you?

How might this awareness affect the next step in your day?

What other things might assist you in **slowing down**?

Take the next step in your day with this practice of **slowing down**. Note your observations and discoveries here.

11

MINDLESS BUSYNESS

*Mindfulness is noticing where
you are, how you are, and simply
that you are, in this moment.*

SPILT MILK

I thought I knew what busy was. Now I have a child and I know busyness in a whole new dimension. Early motherhood is a blur of tiredness, newness, and keeping up with day-by-day developments and changes in my child and her needs. It's so task oriented.

Now looking back, even significant events I thought would be indelibly imprinted on my memory are hard to recall beneath the subsequent layers that followed.

Toddlerhood is another frantic level of adventure. My focus is so outward, keeping up with managing the logistics of the day. Keeping up with, and just ahead of, my adventure mouse, keeping her safe, yet allowing her to stretch her capability as she wobbles along the concrete seawall at our local beach. I'm anticipating the next job ("When I've done this, I need to do that; when I've done that, I'll do . . ."), chasing the unending list just to make it through the day. It's all at such a pace that in my exhaustion and lack of breathing space, I feel like a sleepwalker, zoned out on tiredness, moving through my day on autopilot, a strange mixture of listlessness and urgency.

At times, the moments stretch on, the battles go around and around, and I feel as if we'll be in potty-training mishap land, in hair-washing refusal land, in sticker charts and stuffed toy land forever. In the foreverness of it, I take it for granted, even complain that the day is too this or too that. ("Hurry up and finish swinging so I can go to the supermarket and then get home and get dinner on.") I get through a whole day, feeling like I'm just coping, and then slump onto the couch with a sigh and say "Phewf! Thank goodness the kids are in bed. Perhaps now I can have a moment to myself." Am I missing something as it all rushes slowly by?

Mindfulness

I t can be a challenge to find peace in the busyness of motherhood. Whatever you are doing, it is beneficial to practise connecting with yourself and developing awareness of your being, amongst the thoughts and multiple responsibilities of your day.

The practice here is mindfulness. Mindfulness is an awareness of your being in any moment, an act of being present with what is. In an ashram or monastery, the bells may ring or the gong may sound to call you to mindfulness. As a mother, you can set up your own mindfulness reminders to stop, breathe, and notice where you are, the sensations in your body, your feeling state, and turn your mind toward your experience of being now.

It is easy to get lost in the busyness of your day. A reminder gong on your phone can be an appointment with yourself to practise mindfulness. Small coloured dots placed randomly around the house can be a prompt to stop, breathe, and notice your being. Playing a chant or relaxing music in the evening may help you focus on your inner state as you shepherd your children to bed. An inspiring quote or photo on the fridge can remind you of your daily intention. There are many ways to bring yourself to mindfulness in your journey, as you stand, dutiful audience to slide reruns at the park, wait in traffic, cuddle, console, or sit alongside and listen. Your day will supply other less gentle reminders: the stomp, stomp, stomp of an angry child heading for time out because she won't empty the dishwasher. Play with using these moments as prompts to mindfulness. Irritation, reactivity, or frustration may arise in you. Simply notice them arise and subside, let them bring you into the moment, as it is, where you are, as you are, here and now.

MINDFULNESS: INQUIRY

Practise a moment of mindfulness now. Turn your attention to your awareness. Feel your breath. Notice sensations in your body. Notice your thoughts without judgement; let them arise and subside.

Describe the effect of this moment of mindfulness on you.

Choose a time to practise mindfulness in your mothering day.

What "gong" could you use to remind you to practise in this moment?

Set up a "gong" for yourself in your mothering day today. Note below how you do with this mindfulness practice today and its effect.

12

IS THERE SPACE FOR
ME IN MY LIFE?

*No space in your life to include
yoga? Perhaps yoga can
include your life.*

SPILT MILK

I dash into the supermarket, hurry, hurry! I screech around the aisles, throwing things into my trolley. I have to get home, to the kids, get dinner on, do this, do that. And oh no! A queue! I jog. I jiggle. Wait—this enforced pause is an opportunity. I breathe. *Here I am. I am here.* I practise letting go of the rush and just being here.

Today: a short meditation. Baby woke. I'd usually think, *Drat, there goes my meditation.* But instead of giving up, I bring her through to sit snuggled in my shawl with me. It is so wonderful to share the experience of stillness with her and have her experience this part of my practice. So although my meditation was only seven minutes, I sit with her for another five minutes, and it is beautiful.

When I make the space for meditation in my day, my day is more spacious! My house is messier, but I'm having a better time with my kids. I sit with them more, I play more, I am less stressed and blaming. I feel energised, alive, and perceptive. When they want a story, a cuddle, a drink, I am able to be with them more without the request being "yet another thing I am trying to do in this moment." I still swim around in a swirl of TO DO's and feel a strong impulse to "get up and get on with things," but I hear, *What better thing have you got to do?* and I realise there is no better thing. I am practising being still in myself, feeling spaciousness, fearlessness, connection to my kids and to my inner peace.

Today: I wait in the car for an hour while my daughter does an after-school activity. I have an hour to myself! I do some work and then see an opportunity! I hop into the backseat, fold my legs up, and ahhh, twenty minutes' meditation!

Yoga While Life Continues

Motherhood involves a lot of patience and waiting. Waiting can be frustrating and mind-numbingly boring, or it can be an opportunity to do what you would love to be doing. Wherever you are, you can turn your awareness inside; you can practise yoga. If a half-hour meditation or yoga session is not practical for you in your day, perhaps you can make it up in thirty-second poses, one-minute meditations.

Tadasana, mountain pose, standing upright and grounded, is a fantastic pose while your child takes forever in the public toilet and you stand sentry outside the door. Waiting for your toddler in the bath? Three lovely slow Sun Salutations. Standing by the car while your daughter has a tantrum or brushes her teeth or hunts for her uniform? Tree Pose, Warrior Pose, turning inward to your breath.

The practice here is yoga while life continues. Whatever is going on around you, you can simply focus on your breath. Walking, you can use each step to connect with your inner self: *With this step, I am arriving in this moment; with this step, I am home.* Mantra repetition, *OM*, gives your mind a constant, calming focus while you push the pram or nurse your baby. You can practise hanging-out-the-laundry meditation, practise doing-the-dishes meditation, or practise mindfulness while asking your teenager about her homework intentions.

Practising yoga while life continues will awaken your purpose many times in the day. With a recent top-up of self-connection, you will be more ready in any moment to meet the next thousand moments, more able to tune in, slow down, and rearrange your expectations as necessary.

YOGA WHILE LIFE
CONTINUES: INQUIRY

Name some possible ways you could build **yoga while life continues** into your day today.

Write yourself simple instructions for two different moments.

Try adding these two moments of **yoga while life continues** today. Note here the effect and any discoveries.

Practise **yoga while life continues** two times a day through this week, and mark off each moment below, no matter how small.

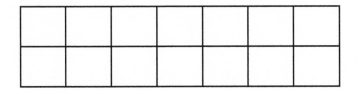

At the end of your week, notice what you did and the effect.

13

HATEFUL HOUSEWORK

What is your true purpose? If it is to be joyously alive in the moment, to be content in your being, then no matter what you are doing, practise pursuit of that purpose.

SPILT MILK

ousework has been a site of inner and outer conflict throughout my life, a cause of fights, fairness, foulness, and fumingness. My housework mantra has been "I hate tidying up after other people."

I feel seethingly victimised by a messy bench someone else could have tidied, a wash still out in the dampening dark as I stagger in the door with my fingers tourniqueted in supermarket bags to cook dinner, only to find my family holidaying blithely around the house.

A friend of mine says "I love wiping surfaces!" as she happily wipes the kitchen bench. What a ludicrously positive frame! Is that all she needs to be happy? How can she so cheerfully accept a life of servitude and meaninglessness? Isn't housework a site of gender politics, aggravation, and resistance? My chore-time is so often spent thinking what else I could be doing, something more worthy of my time and attention. But also I completely get what she means.

I too love a tidy home, a clean bench, a vacuumed, clear, spacious, and ordered room. So why do I hate the task of preparing it? Why don't I love and value the process of getting there?

Embracing my love of these things could transform housework from a site of fury, oppression, litigation, and resentment to one of joy, appreciation, choice, and integration. What will I be giving up if I accept and embrace it? Am I willing to?

What would my new housework mantra of joy and presence be?

Finding Joy in Mundane Tasks

Motherhood is full of mundane and repetitive tasks: wiping walls, floors, bottoms, hands, faces; washing clothes, bodies, bedding, dishes; holding people, books, clothes, half-eaten sandwiches; folding; cleaning; chopping; shopping; waiting; picking up people, toys, scattered clothes; picking them up again . . . and again.

It is worth working on a better relationship with all of these mundane tasks because you live with them intimately. It is no good waiting until it's all done to enjoy your life. No matter what anyone else is doing, you can find joy here and now in any task, even housework! Expect it, accept it, and embrace it.

The practice here is finding joy in mundane tasks. In fact, finding joy is the purpose. You want a clean house, right? Because a clean, orderly house functions well and feels good, it allows you to enjoy your environment. There is an essential joy in each task as an expression of your values, your wishes, your choices. When you engage your purpose, you engage your joy.

"I love a clean bath to bathe my family in!"

"My home is my ashram! I am tidying to create inner peace."

"I will use this time vacuuming to contemplate all the things I appreciate about this house!"

"My home is a living workspace, and I am clearing the floor for the next piece of work!"

"I am so fortunate to be able to shop for wonderful, nourishing food."

With a sense of purpose, you can connect any task in your life to your deepest joy.

FINDING JOY IN MUNDANE TASKS: INQUIRY

Identify two mundane tasks of your mothering week that you find challenging.

What are your current thoughts and approaches to these tasks?

What is the purpose in each of these tasks? What values, wishes, and choices of yours are you expressing by doing them?

What essential joy is there for you in these two tasks?

What new mothering mantra could support you in **finding joy in these mundane tasks**?

Is there anything else you could do to support yourself in developing this approach?

14

SMOOTH PLANS AND BAD BEHAVIOUR

Mothering requires learning on the job. What do we expect of ourselves? We will mess up, and plans will go sideways. What do we expect of ourselves then?

SPILT MILK

If it was at all challenging managing my own life and behaviour, that was mere training for motherhood! Life with kids has been a festival of comic errors and horror stories. Kids throw a spanner in smooth plans all the time; they fill and spill a nappy as I leave the house for that one event that matters, pick prize blooms from sacred gardens, and melt down dramatically at their own birthday parties, especially when mother-in-law attends.

I hope someone laughs when they read that last line, because that just happened to me, so badly. My husband is away, and his mother and sister have come to stay for our daughter's seventh birthday. We slave over labour-intensive party food, plan, cook, clean, and line up the events of the day. I wrangle the gaggle of eight-year-olds as we musical-chair, balloon-game, and pin-the-tail-on-the-donkey. I work my ass off to give my wee girl the best birthday ever. But does she express appreciation? No. Does she behave? Well, yes, spectacularly! But not the way I want her to.

When her spur-of-the-moment call to the trampoline right on food time fails to draw a crowd of followers, she totally derails. She tantrums to new heights and runs away screaming, "This is the worst birthday party EVER!" It is the best demonstration of "ungrateful child" behaviour we could have supplied. It feels like my worst birthday party ever, too.

Have I not brought her up to appreciate the efforts of others? What does it say about me that I cannot control her behaviour? I feel hurt, angry, embarrassed, fearful of judgement. I try to joke about it. Over a well-deserved cuppa, I confess to my discomfort. I read judgement in my mother-in-law's silence. How swiftly I jump to my child's actions being a reflection of my own worth.

Adjusting Expectations

Smooth plans and mothering often don't go together. You may not meet every plan change as well as you wish. In fact, you definitely will not. Motherhood is a training in flexibility and detachment. As a mother, you are responsible for many things, getting people places on time, fed, dressed, prepared for life. It just so happens life will not comply, no matter how well you prepare. It's not just seven-year-olds who have a fantasy in their head of what a successful party is and who believe everyone should also have that picture and act accordingly; mothers do too!

You will get plenty of opportunities to practise accepting reality and letting go of trying to control life. It's not your fault that you cannot change the weather, or mind-control others, so don't go there. Blame and shame will only suck you deeper into the swamp of delusion that it is up to you to keep everyone happy.

The practice here is adjusting expectations. Notice what is, accept that you are doing your best and cannot control the universe, and then adjust your expectations to a more generous understanding. Expectations are tricky in the first place; they cut across the reality of what is unfolding.

Some realities in this instance are: (1) parties are high-pressure events, (2) real life does not comply with perfect pictures of what will happen, (3) mothers' pictures often don't include an ungrateful child, (4) seven-year-olds aren't renowned for seeing or appreciating the work that their mothers and others do making life happen well for them, (5) that can hurt, and (6) you are all doing your best, mother-in-law included.

ADJUSTING EXPECTATIONS: INQUIRY

What smooth plans have you had go sideways recently? What happened?

How did you respond?

What were your expectations?

What were the realities of the situation?

What understanding would you like to cultivate in such a moment?

What adjustment might you make to your expectations today?

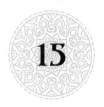

15

I'M SO OVER THIS

How you respond to each situation, each moment, moves you toward or away from living your life as you want to live it. This is the moment you are living now. There is no other time; there is no better time.

SPILT MILK

I t's not all hard yards, but perseverance is big in my life at the moment. I have many moments of wonderment: dancing with the girls, wonderment at their language, seeing their wonderment at the world, and being amazed at their even being, and mine. But I am so "in" motherhood, there is a lack of time to reflect, a lack of time to stock-take, to progress, to feel and develop a sense of attainment. I find myself trying to get out of where I am, to get to the next place, the next task, the next conversation, the next room, the next time, trying to get time to do something else. I am not living the preciousness of each moment.

Early motherhood is a total immersion experience. I am climbed on at every moment, demanded of, picked at, fiddled with, dribbled on, tapped for attention, scratched, sucked, and pulled. Someone always needs to be carried, cuddled, held, or breastfed. I walk for back-aching weeks crouched like a gibbon, a human Zimmer frame overhanging my on-the-cusp-of-walking toddler. At times, it drives me crazy; I want to shout, "Leave me alone!" Looking back ten years later, I wonder at the irony of it: now I'm lucky if I get a cuddle without asking.

My ten-year-old still wants me to walk her to school. I have tried all sorts of tactics to encourage her to do it alone. Surely, at ten, she should be doing this independently and happily like other kids. But she isn't. My brother-in-law says, "Oh, I miss it! Make the most of it! It'll pass. Walk her to school for as long as she wants." Really? I've been pushing things along, trying to create more space. But it's not forever, is it? It is now. What a liberating approach, to just do it and love what it is while I can. So today, I just do it and really enjoy it. We hold hands down the hill. We chat. I feel this time as a gift.

Having the Time of Your Life While You're Having It

In mother-time, the days are long and the years short. Time measures differently from a working day or project cycle; there are no set hours, no crisp start and finish, no "motherhood—done," tick! The infant and toddler years are so consuming and the developments so incremental that it can be hard to see changes without time lapse. When you can't feel change and the experience is total immersion day in and day out, it is hard to be mindful that things won't always be like this.

The saying "You don't know what you've got till it's gone" is testimony to our tendency to take the blessings of the moment for granted. If you find yourself wishing time away or looking forward to "the time when . . ." or "being on the other side of . . ." know that that time will come. This time will most definitely melt away, but look closely or you could miss it in the intensity. This is the only time to have the experience in front of you. This is the time of your life, and you are in it now.

The practice here is having the time of your life while you're having it. This practice is an antidote to wishful thinking and regret, and a foothold for satisfaction. To celebrate the experience of where you are is to embrace what may feel repetitive, but know it to be a unique moment, to feel this cuddle, this walk, what is alive and new in this moment, this day. Yes, there will be challenges, but don't wish time away. This is the time of your life. The present is not to be tolerated; it is to be loved as it is, valued for what it is. There is joy and liberation in living the life you have while you have it. Embrace this time. It will pass.

HAVING THE TIME OF YOUR LIFE WHILE YOU'RE HAVING IT: INQUIRY

What aspects of your life as a mother are you treasuring today?

What aspects of your life as a mother are you struggling with today?

How do you respond to these treasures and struggles?

If you consider **having the time of your life while you are having it**, how might you respond differently?

What could assist you in having the time of your life today?

What might prevent you having the time of your life today?

When you come across a moment of treasure or struggle in your day today, practise being exactly where you are in your life. Breathe; bring your awareness to this moment. It is enough. Note down what occurs when you practise **having the time of your life while you're having it**.

16

INVISIBLE WORK

*When you are focused on the
purpose of knowing the self,
then every act, every task, no
matter how grand or small,
is equally important. In
every moment, you have the
opportunity to attain peace,
to attain happiness
and contentment.*

SPILT MILK

As a mother, I work harder than ever, learn more than ever, doing work I know is the most valuable I could ever hope to do. Yet why do I feel so unsatisfied in myself? Why does my life as a mother feel so full of drudgery? When I get through difficult days well, even REALLY well, when I engage thoughtfully with parenting and mothering issues, achieve excellence in problem-solving, human relations, and time management, why do I feel so unrecognised? Perhaps because nobody recognises it! I didn't become a mother for the recognition, but I'm working really hard here and I feel undervalued.

My newborn and toddler are unable to say "Mum, you did that really well: you managed to look after the needs of three people, grocery shop, nappy change, feed, put to sleep, toilet train, respect, coach, dress, tidy, cook, clean, read to, consider healthy eating options, encourage, manage your own feelings of frustration, provide excellent attention, and LOVE us through it all, ALL before lunchtime. You are doing a great job, Mum." Words that would mean a lot at times when all I feel at the end of the day is sleep deprived, tired of looking after others, and conscious of how little I have "achieved." I live in an achievement culture. This is hard.

In other circumstances, work of this quality would gain me a raise or a promotion; at the very least, I'd be paid. But what value does five years of full-time mothering add to my CV? Mothering is untrained, invisible, crucial, ignored, disruptive; it is at once so important and so nebulous. I am caught in a social conflict. Is mothering the most important social investment I could ever make or the least productive of occupations? It is hard to feel the value of my efforts and time.

Valuing Your Choice

All mothers are working. Let's get that clear for a start. Whether you choose to work at home full-time with the important task of raising your children or work elsewhere at an office, lecture theatre, laboratory, surgery, or salon, whether you pay others to look after your kids while you go out to work or have the support of family in minding them, or whether you work at your own projects from home, juggling domestic chores with professional tasks, you are working. There is no "right" way to reconcile career, home, and motherhood; there is only what is right for you.

How you think and feel about your circumstances and choices will make a difference to how you think and feel about yourself as a mother. If you are working at home, raising your children as your main job, the remuneration, status, and professional identity that often signal value and reward time and effort will be missing from the picture. If this anomaly in the mothering and value equation leaves you feeling a deficit, reflecting on the heart of your choices will help you toward finding your balance.

The practice here is valuing your choice. Being conscious of what choices you are making and why creates alignment between your choices and what matters to you. It empowers you to make purposeful adjustments so that your choices support your intention and their value is clear.

You are the one who shapes your choices; you are the one who shapes your life. To be conscious and responsible for your choices paves the journey to self-knowledge.

VALUING YOUR CHOICE: INQUIRY

What choices have you made about how you are "doing" motherhood?

Why did you make these choices?

What do you value most about what comes from these choices?

What do you find challenging that comes from these choices?

What would you like to adjust in how you are "doing" the job of mothering?

Choose one. If you made one small step toward this today, what would it be?

17

I USED TO BE SUCCESSFUL: WORK AND WORTH

What does it mean to be truly successful? Is it winning at golf, being lucrative in business, or being swift at speed-reading? What good are these things if you do not succeed at being content with your life?

SPILT MILK

Motherhood is a world of human worth beyond commercial value or social status. It capsizes the notions of success I've been measured by and measure with. I'm used to feeling successful or at least recognised in my professional identity. Approval, achievement, recognition, status, and visibility have added to my sense of success and self-worth.

I made the choice to have children. I want to be with them through these early years to give them the best start in life. I believe I am the best person to give them the daily love and care I want for them and that they need in order to thrive. I've chosen this. I know it is up to me to recognise and value the time, energy, and work I do raising my children, but I am in a profound state of conflict. Is motherhood career death or the most important work I could ever hope to do? I get plenty of outer signs of the first and not many to the second. But what do I think? My success markers are adrift.

I'm trying to keep my career going, to activate and create, stay productive, continue with "my life." But with motherhood, there's no PAUSE; it's hard to write an email with someone hanging off my arm and shouting for attention. So for my sanity, I have put my two-year-old in one morning of care, and now I'm supposed to be doing some "real work."

I know motherhood is real work. Demanding and unpaid, but humanly valuable like no other job. In the absence of social recognition, I will have to back myself, stand up for this thing I am putting my all into. Beyond keeping them alive, sheltered, fed, and loved, success in motherhood to me is being alongside now, investing in a quality relationship with my children, supporting their developing sense of who they are in the world. I am banking on collecting my reward in daily satisfaction and in part payments over the rest of my life.

Recognising Success

Mothering is work. It is a job. But it is hard to assess how good a job you're doing. One day, you're nailing it; the next, it's nailing you.

From yummy mummy to executive superwoman, social messages abound about what makes a successful mother. There is pressure to go out to work and earn, pressure to stay home and look after your child, and pressure to do both simultaneously. In a culture where work, pay, and worth go together, it is a challenge to feel the human value of the endeavour of motherhood as reward enough. However you navigate it, on what do you base your day-to-day sense of success as a mother?

The practice here is recognising success. It is important to orient yourself to the value of what you do and recognise your success in the course of the day. To *re-cognise* is literally to re-understand, to consciously affirm your moments of success as a mother and why they are important to you.

You choose your measure of success. Got your kids into the car well under trying circumstances? Shopped and made a meal? Made time to read to your eleven-year-old? Got yourself to bed before ten p.m.? Great! Well done! You know these things are important. Recognise success when it happens. Acknowledge your success: say it out loud, or even better, let your child, partner, or friend know what you've succeeded at and why it matters.

I have succeeded in making space to walk you to school. It matters to me that I take your distress about drop-off seriously. Success to me as a mother is acting on your concerns in this moment.

RECOGNISING SUCCESS: INQUIRY

What does "success" as a mother mean to you?

What do you do in order to be successful as a mother?

Write out a moment of success from your mothering day, no matter how small. Include what you did that was successful, why it mattered to you, and how you know that you were successful.

When do you feel most successful as a mother? Why?

Name your three core strengths as a mother.

18

HOW DO I
ACHIEVE
ANYTHING?

*Our goal in life is not to get
over the finish line first, then
ask, "Did I live as I wanted?"
Life is in the journey, not
the destination. Ask yourself
now: "What is important to
me to achieve in life?"*

SPILT MILK

My first midwife tells me of her mother saying, "I always had my nappies washed and on the line by ten a.m." She seems to think it a laughable goal, exposing subservience, a pitiable housewife prioritizing menial tasks as signifiers of her achievement. But the funny thing is, the comment stays with me, and as I also use cloth nappies for my baby, I find myself feeling deeply satisfied when I get them out on the line before ten a.m. So I begin to make it a goal, and it is one of the few things in the early days that gives me a sense of accomplishment.

I'm not sure I was a stress bunny before I had kids. I experienced anxiety and stress at times, but it wasn't like this. Simultaneously meeting the expectations of a career and motherhood has firmly secured my tendency to rush from task to task. Even sitting still (when does that happen?), I am burning adrenaline.

I feel time-poor for doing things for me, my mind, myself, and walk instead in the zombie-glue of hours spent attendant to someone else's life and learning. It is hard to reconcile my previously accelerating achievement frame with the otherworldly slowness of mothering, this glacially-paced, all-consuming existence. How do I achieve anything?

I love my kids; I am super interested in what they are doing; I'm never bored of them. I love the cuddles, the games, the sight of them sleeping, eating, playing. I love being there, being the one who is there for them. But I struggle with giving over my time and self so fully to someone else. My old ambition is thwarted. It's a strange contradiction, so urgent and so slow.

Achievement Satisfaction

Flat-out but never finished? Piles of washing, toys, dishes, things to wipe up, clean, and tidy everywhere you look? Rushing home from after-school activities to cook dinner, get the wash in, bear witness to homework and guitar practice, via the supermarket, salon, mammogram clinic, chemist, and petrol station? And still no sense of real achievement?

The satisfaction that comes with well-defined achievement can be lost in the repetitive operational missions of a mothering day. The small victory of a clean kitchen doesn't clearly contribute to a lifetime's cumulative value. But satisfaction does.

The practice here is achievement satisfaction, collecting rewards from your daily achievements. Satisfaction of a job well done is accumulative and readily on hand in the unceasing business of mothering. Of course there is always more to do, and you don't just pick up toys or clean the kitchen once. But when you appreciate achievement, no matter how small, you can collect satisfaction as you go. That's what *appreciation* means: growing the value of something. Each task holds the sweet satisfaction of achievement if you can sew, reap, and savour it.

Try these strategies: Take the task in front of you. Identify the task purpose: *I will make this phone call in order to create peace of mind.* Acknowledge real tasks—dressing a toddler counts! Acknowledge each part of a larger task: *Cook dinner* is made up of *find recipe, grocery shop, harvest garden vegetables, put rice on . . .* naming the achievement of each part increases the number of opportunities for achievement satisfaction in your day. Define: *I will tidy for twenty minutes then stop.* Set your lowest bar for satisfaction: *Kitchen clear enough to cook the next meal.* Small change adds up. Then collect the satisfaction of each small achievement.

ACHIEVEMENT SATISFACTION: INQUIRY

Take a task that lies ahead in your mothering day. What is the purpose of this task?

Break it down into its smaller parts, each with a start and a finish.

Take one part. What is the purpose of this task?

What is your lowest bar for satisfaction in achieving this task?

When you complete the task, pause, collect your satisfaction, and savour it. Note your experience here.

As you go through your day, practise identifying the satisfaction available in achieving each task. Then pause, collect, and savour it.

19

RELENTLESS WONDERFULNESS

*Thank you for mama being
born, and for borning us.*
—Ava, age 6

SPILT MILK

L ife in my house is one constant roleplay. Fairies, butterflies, princesses, and mermaids are constantly rummaging in the dress-up box, doing inventive things with tiaras, tissues, and bits of fabric. We have regulars: Bamboo who wears the pink plastic clippy-clop shoes and skids dangerously on the wooden floor but WILL NOT take off those darn shoes. There's Curtsey in the white and pink ruffle dress, Bow who spends a lot of time on her phone, and also Butterfly, Flower, and occasionally Rainbow. They introduce themselves and visit for tea parties, make playdough cakes, paint, dance to "Swamp Lake," and do award-winning shows with ten-minute curtain calls for an audience. I am that audience.

It is creative and brilliantly funny. Every day, I laugh so hard, stifling giggles when my two-year-old erupts into the swimming show, hair scuffed up and steamy goggles squashing eyes askew. I belly-laugh in the Little Red Riding Hood show performed inexplicably in faux "Japanese" by puppets with extreme neck angles who make brief and blazing entrances then mutter at eyebrow height in the quivering puppet tent.

It is wonderful and hilarious, and I believe play is an essential part of healthy human development, but I really have so many other things to do. It sounds so terrible, but sometimes I end up tolerating hours of play with my children when the truth is I am so sick of watching yet another show, being the voice of some animal or other, rolling playdough, pretending to eat biscuits made of sand. I'm sure I'm not the best playmate, stewing in frustration and boredom, feeling pressure to play along. How can I say "no"? Isn't this my job? Isn't this a golden chance to enhance my children's lives by being alongside them?

Patience with the Journey

The Dalai Lama tells the story of being on a long haul flight with a young family. Eventually, the active toddler and dad are exhausted and fall asleep. The mother stays up with the unsettled baby. Hours later, the Dalai Lama wakes and realises that the mother has not slept at all. He is amazed at her capacity for patience, that she is still caring, still devoted to the welfare of her children. "For myself, I simply cannot imagine being so patient!" he says. And that's the Dalai Lama talking!

Being a mother is tiring, delightful, demanding, worrisome, fascinating, and much, much more. It often requires that you make sacrifices, putting aside your own needs, though your innards may scream for rest, for some quiet, to walk unencumbered, to have a break, to do your own thing. You are a person with your own needs, and sometimes they conflict with the job of being a mother. That's the rub of the mothering journey. What do you cultivate in response to it?

The practice here is patience with the journey. As with a trip to the dentist, you are more able to tolerate short-term pain if you hold the long-term purpose of healthy teeth in mind. Similarly, with motherhood, the patience required to tolerate tiredness, repetitive story-book boredom syndrome, and staying steady during the most spectacular of tantrums is strengthened in the context of your larger journey, your values, your choices, and your greater purpose. Knowing your purpose contextualises fleeting compromise and helps foster patience with yourself, with your children, and with the journey of motherhood.

PATIENCE WITH THE JOURNEY: INQUIRY

Let's have a look at the big picture. Write the brief story of your choice to become a mother, your hopes, your motivation, what happened, and what you have learned.

What do you appreciate when you reflect on your journey so far?

Where are you at currently in your journey as a mother; what are you are asking, learning, and appreciating?

Where are you cultivating *santosha*, contentment, acceptance of what is, of yourself and of others? What are you learning about it?

Imagine, far in the future, you are reflecting back on your mothering journey. What do you imagine is precious to you about it? What do you appreciate from this perspective?

PART THREE

Tapas

SELF-DISCIPLINE

20

MAD, BAD, AND SAD
MOTHERING MOMENTS

*We have to journey through the
light and the dark; there is no
way around it.*

SPILT MILK

I n a moment of frustration about cleaning the rabbit hutch, I snatch the scrubbing brush from my daughter. I burst and snatch. I do the thing I say not to. Immediately, I feel bad. I feel childish. I don't feel equipped to be a mother at all. It is a bad mothering moment. This is not how I want to be as a mother.

Perhaps I can get some value from this moment and use it to investigate and learn from. I sit and contemplate. I feel disturbed, ashamed, bad, and guilty. Guilt is knowing I did wrong and feeling powerless to change it. Shame is embarrassment that my faults are revealed, a judgement that I am flawed. I feel a dent in my heart.

So what happened? I said, "No DVD until you've cleaned the rabbit hutch," but I didn't hold the line. I undermined my own boundary. Then I blamed my daughter and deferred responsibility by nagging: "I've been asking you to clean the rabbit hutch all morning . . ." Then I felt powerless, so I tried to reassert my authority by snatching. What can I learn here? Being a mother is requiring me to practise being clearer. It is my job to be the adult, to set boundaries and stick to them.

What a piece of work it is to drop guilt and move forward! I don't want to be stuck here going over my failures and faults. I have to apply my will and learn what to do differently. This moment is a very clear example of how I undermine a boundary, blame someone else, and then snap. I want to do better than this.

I rehearse a clearer script: "I've asked you to clean the rabbit hutch. If you haven't started in five minutes, there will be no DVD today. I will set the timer starting now." Now both of our jobs are clear, the consequence is clear, and I know what line to hold.

Embracing the Light and the Dark

Your relationship with your children is a mirror of your relationship to yourself. You will not always be the self you want the world to see. Mothering will challenge every aspect of your behaviour. Everything you thought you had a grip on or had smoothed over will be tilled to the surface. You will meet the light and the dark: your fear of not belonging, your desire to control others, your habit of trying to keep everyone happy at your own expense . . . The list of challenges to your sense of self will be boundless. The heat of these challenges provides an opportunity to burn off the dross. This is *tapas*: the purifying fire of self-discipline.

The practice here is embracing the light and the dark. Everyone has their own journey, their own discomforts, anxieties, and celebrations. This is yours. You will respond as you do. You will do something old or something new, something clumsy, upsetting, or less than perfect. The lessons are tailor made to you. Your journey is your responsibility, your gift, your opportunity. That old soil freshly turned is fertile ground for what you want to cultivate. Motherhood is illuminating, a worthy journey. Embrace the light and the dark of it.

You are doing your best at seeking and cultivating self-knowledge. Damning judgement is not conducive to learning. No matter how old or squirmy the discomfort of a bad mothering moment, embrace your journey and your learning. Apply your conscious mind to your learning. Ask, *What do I learn from this? What could I do differently next time?* Be compassionate and encouraging. Tell yourself, *I am doing my best at learning to do something new. I will keep going!*

EMBRACING THE LIGHT AND THE DARK: INQUIRY

Describe a recent mad, sad, or bad mothering moment you experienced.

What was your intention in this moment?

What did you doubt or fear in this moment?

What learning is available to you from this?

What could you do differently next time?

What encouragement can you give yourself that acknowledges the value of **embracing the light and the dark** in your mothering journey?

21

BEING MORE THAN MYSELF

Having a partner is one thing, but no matter how close and intimate, having a child is quite different. No other relationship is like it.

SPILT MILK

The instant my first baby was born, that was it; I was never, ever, just me again. I was two people, and now I am three. I am primarily responsible for three lives. I live in three places at any moment, with three people's intimate experiences in my heart. I hold my children in my being with the same concern I have for myself. No significant decision made after the moment I gave birth has ever been about just me. Even insignificant decisions—whether to stop at the supermarket, what to cook, when to book an appointment, when to go to bed—are not just about me anymore.

I was not prepared for the depth of nature's conquest over my individuality. Perhaps I thought the intense bond was optional, but it isn't. I'm hardwired for it. It doesn't mean I know what I'm doing, though. There is no instinct for folding cloth nappies or knowing whether to give paracetamol.

The innate biology of motherhood has me welling with panic when my three-year-old disappears in the department store or when my fifteen-year-old isn't home from the party by midnight as agreed. My mother-animal instinct kicks in with vivid imaginings of what's gone wrong. Knotty adrenaline urges me to act in getting to and protecting my child. Then when I find my three-year-old hiding gleefully in a rack of clothes or my fifteen-year-old home at 12:25 but out at the gate kissing a boy with her phone in her back pocket on silent, I am both relieved and furious.

I want to hold her and shout at her at the same time. She's safe, but I still have my surging guts to deal with. My brain stem battles my frontal cortex. Weighing powerful biology against better judgement complicates things, and I'm left wound up and confused.

Love and Accept Your Humanity

What do you have in common with a lioness defending her cubs, a crocodile with a tender mouthful of hatchlings, and an oystercatcher faking a broken wing to lure intruders away from her nest? You are all animals programmed to protect your offspring. Your successful biology requires you to have the same vigilant level of concern for yourself and your children. Add the stressors of sleep deprivation, hormonal sensitivity, toddler escapes, teenage emotions, social pressures, and the demands of managing additional lives, and you multiply the chances of your brain stem giving you shots of full-throttle fight, flight, or freeze in any given day.

You are also a forward-thinking, aspirational, consequence-predicting, data-processing, frontal lobe–carrying animal with a powerful mind that collates history, culture, stories, memories, and information. At times you will feel torn between your impulse to react and your choice to act toward an enlightened outcome. There is no shame in this dilemma; it is an inescapable and vital part of being human. *Tapas*, meet motherhood.

The practice here is love and accept your humanity. You cannot discount your brain stem; you can only work with it. Spiritual teachers through the ages acknowledge it takes discipline and practice to convert our base human responses into more sophisticated ones that will benefit ourselves and our communities. Anger, jealousy, depression, anxiety, and panic all have roots in the brain stem, but to fight, flee, or freeze in response to them is to stay trapped there. To love and accept your humanity, to feel your vulnerability and that of those around you, is a principal component in the inner work of motherhood.

LOVE AND ACCEPT YOUR
HUMANITY: INQUIRY

Identify a recent mothering incident where you reacted instinctively. Note what you appreciate about your response.

Identify a current or recent mothering incident of struggle between reacting and making a considered response. What can you appreciate about this struggle?

Identify a recent mothering incident where you made a considered response. Describe the process you went through to enable this response and its effect.

What love and acceptance are you waking to in the humanity of your mothering journey?

Where could you apply this awareness in your day ahead?

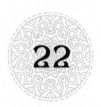

22

BLAME

*Blame keeps us trapped in the idea
that someone else is responsible for
our life. Taking responsibility means
freeing ourselves to experience the
joy we yearn for.*

SPILT MILK

I feel blaming. My husband didn't consult me about taking time away. I am upset. I feel he is having a good life at my expense. After all, *I* can't just drop the kids and go off without telling him. What about *me*?! I accuse him of relying thoughtlessly on me and taking me for granted. I blame him for not doing this hard work of mothering for me, for not looking after me, for having a better life than me. I feel powerless, unappreciated, hurt, angry.

There is a cost to me in this blame. The cost of blame is fights, friction, distance, discomfort. It does no good for me to blame myself, my husband, or the world for my feelings of dissatisfaction. It does me no good to blame my children for my choice to stay home with them. Blaming others for my feelings gives me no advantage.

I feel I have no choice. I feel consumed and submerged in the role of mothering. I blame myself for being tied to my desire to be the best mother I can.

What is the work in front of me? What do I need to do? I need to take more responsibility for myself. I need to nourish and uplift myself. Burnout and blowout is not useful to me or my family. I need to heal this old resentful story about being oppressed by motherhood.

What could I gain from this? I want to learn how to act more responsibly for myself. I am responsible for my own happiness.

I could identify when I need time away BEFORE I need it. I could understand more about what I want for myself, plan time for me, arrange childcare, and practise making my times apart from my children easier.

Taking Responsibility

Blame emerges in response to feeling hurt, frightened, judged, fearful of being rejected, of not getting enough love, of not meeting expectations, your own or others'. Blame is adversarial, argumentative, and oppositional. Blaming displaces responsibility and puts the power to determine your happiness into the hands of others. Blaming others apportions too much influence and power to someone else. Blaming yourself assumes you have too much control over something you cannot change, or enslaves you in reliving the past, reinforcing thoughts of yourself as stupid, ignorant, shameful, or guilty. Blame holds you in old victim stories, plots revenge and retaliation, picks at old wounds of humiliation. Blame keeps you weak and dependent. So what is the antidote to this ancient drama?

The practice here is taking responsibility. Being responsible, response-able, means engaging your strength, your resilience and will, and giving the lead to the part of you that is able to respond with something new. Taking responsibility enables you to cultivate the wisdom that comes alive even in painful situations. This is *tapas*: persevering in the heat of the cleansing fire!

This is not time to dwell on your faults. Taking or making blame is unlikely to create the response you want to have in this situation. Now is the time to invest in forgiveness, steadiness, liberation, and self-containment. Let go of the desire to find fault. Hold onto understanding and wisdom. Increase your capacity to respond afresh, to now. What other response would you like to cultivate? What response will create the love, connection, joy, and liberation you long for?

TAKING RESPONSIBILITY: INQUIRY

Do you experience blame in your life as a mother? How does the story of this blame go?

Who do you think is responsible for creating this situation?

What does this blame grow in you?

Is that really what you want to choose? What other responses would you like to choose in this situation? (Blame is sneaky; look out for words of revenge.)

Choose one of these new responses. If you took responsibility to enact this, how might a new story of this situation go?

What new ideas are occurring to you about **taking responsibility**?

How might you practise this in your day today?

23

ANXIETY, WORRY, FEAR, AND OVERWHELM

You are no good worried; your worry adds nothing; your worry offers nothing to your family. Your peace offers a lot; your peace adds a lot. Do everything you can to build peace. You are here now. You are here.

SPILT MILK

I have felt over the last few weeks a pain in my solar plexus when I am anxious, rushing, bustling my children in, around, and out of the supermarket, into and out of the car, into and out of the house, rushing . . . I need to stop. I need to change this mode of operating.

An opportunity comes to go on a four-day retreat. To go feels like a big deal. I have been keeping such a tight grip on my family life—school activities, boundaries and budgets, working and shopping—that I find I'm like a tight-gripped hand, frozen, immobilised into a stiff, numb shape. After so long, it is hard to let go.

Why am I so reluctant? Deep down, I believe I cannot and should not leave my kids, that they might not be okay without me, that I need to be here for . . . what? To make afternoon tea, wash, clean, be there. *Really?* It is shocking to see how much doing an excellent job of mothering is overriding my choice to have time off the treadmill. After some painful creaking and releasing, I uncurl my hibernating "retreat taker" within. I need to practise flexibility. I go.

I'm in the car. I'm on the plane. I'm in the taxi. I'm at the retreat.

I call home. My youngest child is sick. I am agitated, anxious. I want to control how my husband looks after her, to instruct, to be kept up to date. I call again the next day. It's hard to hear in all the noise; my little one is crying, my big girl is shouting "DANCING QUEEN" at the top of her lungs. Through the racket, my husband tells me our wee girl vomited twice yesterday, still has diarrhoea. It is totally disturbing. "Don't worry," he hollers, then the phone cuts out.

I am worried. I am anxious. I wish I hadn't called. I feel torn, upset. I try to tell myself, *You are off duty. Care is being taken. Let care be taken of you.*

Honour Your Self

Broken sleep, rushing pulse, erratic breathing, feeling unfocused, irritable, easily fatigued, digestive problems, a general feeling of panic, headaches . . . symptoms of stress and anxiety. If this is your experience of motherhood, you will not be enjoying it. It is important to develop some balance, some new habits, some space and calm. Getting off the whizzing treadmill and slowing things down is a challenge when everything is moving at such a pace.

Being late, a flat tyre, a messy house, resistant children, a crayon drawing on the wall: these are the spilt milk, the things that happen outside you. Feelings of panic at being late, worry at the flat tyre, overwhelm at the prospect of tidying your house, frustration mobilizing reluctant kids, anger at the unwanted home decorating: these are your internal responses to the spilt milk. What happens inside you is where the stress occurs.

The good news is that you can choose other responses. It takes discipline to direct your energy purposefully in the heat of your anxiety, worry, fear, and overwhelm, but it is possible. It takes practice, time, and consciousness, but you can do it. You are feeling the burn of *tapas*. As uncomfortable as it is, motherhood is offering you the opportunity to cultivate peace, contentment, and steadiness.

The practice here is honour your self. Name your anxiety, identify your concerns, understand the thoughts with which you create your suffering, and get alongside yourself with less judgement and more acceptance. From this place, it is possible to choose a more joyous and liberating response to those outside stressors. A five-minute retreat for self-inquiry and contemplation will honour and support you in your journey. Remember, the mountain is climbed in many small steps, and each small step counts.

HONOUR YOUR SELF: INQUIRY

Recall a recent mothering moment where you experienced anxiety, worry, fear, or overwhelm. Describe what was happening externally.

What was happening internally? What did you . . .
. . . think?

. . . feel?

. . . do?

Tune into yourself now. Sit, close your eyes, breathe in deep and out long a couple of times. Ask yourself, *What does this mothering moment hold for me?* and note what arises.

Now ask, *What more should I know about this mothering moment?*

That is all you need to do for now. There is no need to rush onto the next thing. Accept and value that you are on a journey and this is where you are right now. **Honour your self.**

24

RESENTMENT
AND NEGATIVITY

*To make progress, each new
step must leave behind the
last.*

SPILT MILK

Today, being at home with preschoolers is like walking in glue. I cannot get anything worthwhile done! I do 1001 mundane things, make beds, prep food, wash, dress, wipe, cuddle, listen, play, clean, and do it all again, but I have no sense of achievement.

I feel trapped and bored. I resent my situation. I feel like this time at home is limiting my career. I feel the pressure of jobs I don't need to do. I feel victimised by the pile of junk in the corner of the bedroom. I snap at my kids, then feel guilty.

Negativity monologues in my head: *I have to endure this burden, wasting my energy on the time-guzzling duties and activities of mothering and housework. Imagine what other wonderful, important things I could be doing! What will others think of me? Has it ruined my career? Having kids has limited my potential!*

I'm putting a lot of energy into holding onto this negative story that doesn't serve me well. I need another script! One that unhooks me from viewing this time as unfair somehow. This is what I have, and it is wonderful. I chose to be a mother. I would choose it again. The drudgery is challenging, but I'm committed to it, so I need to let that negative stuff go and give myself something better to hold onto.

My expectations about what I "achieve" in my day are limiting my experience of my day and creating anxiety. I want to let go of those expectations. I want to hold onto the joy, abundance, and love in my life. I want to hold onto the value of my journey, to forgiveness, patience, and appreciation for what I have, to good company, to clear boundaries, to being present with my children and myself in the moment, to what I love in being a mother.

Holding On and Letting Go

To move, whether it's walking, a yoga pose, or inner progress, you need to know what to let go of and what to hold onto. Energizing one area and relaxing another are two different actions but both part of the same movement. Yoga requires intention, discipline, and practice.

This discipline extends to your inner yoga; it helps to be clear about what you want to hold onto and what you want to let go of. Being intentional in your inner posture toward something means you are anchored to your developing inner strength and flexibility. This also takes practice.

The practice here is knowing what to let go of and what to hold onto. Like climbing a ladder, each rung must be released in order to grasp the next.

Experiences are reinforced by how we interpret them. If they are translated through outdated ideas, old prejudices, and judgements, that is what they will reinforce. Every moment is an opportunity to let go of old notions that do not serve you and hold more firmly to the joy and freedom you are pursuing.

Knowing what you are letting go of and holding onto enables you to respond more purposefully to who and what is in front of you. In murky moments, knowing what you are holding onto and letting go of will enable you to move forward consciously in your living and being.

HOLDING ON AND
LETTING GO: INQUIRY

Identify a current situation in your mothering life you are finding unclear, murky, or challenging.

What has been your response so far?

What do you want to hold onto more firmly in your life as a
mother?

What do you need to let go of in order to do this?

How might this apply to the situation you have identified?

Now take a minute to close your eyes, picture yourself in the
situation, and practise being intentional with what you are holding onto and letting go of. Note here what is awakening in you.

25

WHEN IT'S
SOMEONE ELSE'S
FAULT

*Forgiveness is a constant act;
recommit to it in every new
moment.*

SPILT MILK

We're driving north for a family holiday when inexplicably from the curve of traffic, a car pulls out, accelerating straight toward us. I can do nothing to stop it. I think, *This can't be happening.* It happens. Incredible, soul-punching impact. My being screams internally, *NO! NOT YET! MY KIDS!* Powerful g-forces pitch us sideways. I expect blackness, but all goes white. Airbags. Smoke. I can't see. I'm winding the steering wheel futilely trying to correct the violent metal-grinding spin. I need to reach my kids, three and six years old, in the back, to connect and reassure. In the chaos, I hear my voice, steady and clear, calling, "We're okay . . . we're still okay . . . we're still okay . . ." because for every millisecond more until the next thing happens, we are okay, okay in this suspended arc of elasticated time, *we are still okay* . . . The car lurches to a stop. My eyes meet my husband's as we turn . . . and there they are, our daughters, alive. Amid shattered glass and toys, alive. We wrench doors open, climb out. My husband does a jubilant dance in the road: "The ABS brakes worked; the seatbelts worked! We're alive." I shout down the road, "You BASTARD!" We scoop in, each clutch a child. Alive. Alive. Stumble shaking to the roadside. I've pissed myself in the impact. My neck hurts. People come running. Alive.

I had a lot of work to do to forgive that man. He lied to police, refused restorative justice, left the country to avoid consequences. I wanted him to face the hurt, pain, and fear his carelessness cost us. One day, meditating on forgiveness, an aurora borealis of ribbon streams skyward from my heart; I let go of fault-finding and feel deep gratitude, for my practice, for my life, for all I have, even for the accident, which is teaching me to forgive. I'm drawing it out of myself, now and now and now again. I realise forgiveness is an ongoing act.

Forgiveness of Others

Motherhood is the most personal, familial, intimate, and important of journeys. It stirs passionate emotions and primitive reactions. When you have been hurt, wronged, offended, or rejected, when someone has impacted your life adversely, it is tempting to retaliate. It is tempting to seek revenge, to hit back, punish, and return the pain, or to vindicate your suffering and prove that you have been wronged. However, committing to this path can be as harmful as the original wound. Focusing your energy and time on your distress can entrap you in hours of negative storytelling, reliving and reinforcing your trauma and grief.

The practice here is forgiveness. Forgiveness frees you from the impact another person has to negatively affect your life or rob you of the joy that is rightfully yours. Forgiveness is an act of reclaiming your power to choose to live your life in love and freedom. Forgiveness is not a victim state; quite the opposite. It is a process of empowerment, a refusal to sink into the dark, and a commitment to carry yourself to the light. It takes time, willpower, and strength to lift yourself above the mire and draw your intention toward receiving the good in and around you.

To forgive, you must create the conditions in which you can focus on what is good. Consider which people, places, and ideas in your day encourage and enable forgiveness and which don't. If you find yourself getting caught in hurt, turn your attention toward the life you are creating, to choosing happiness, to taking responsibility for your choices. Forgiveness is a constant act, moment by moment, day by day, an ongoing commitment to living your own wisdom, joy, and purpose.

FORGIVENESS OF OTHERS: INQUIRY

If there is someone or something you want to forgive, name what you are choosing to forgive. (If this inquiry feels too big, practise with little things; the process is the same.)

What benefit do you see for yourself in forgiving this?

What could you forgive yourself of in this situation?

In order to forgive, what will you need to let go of?

What are you choosing to create in its place?

What things could you do in your mothering day to strengthen your commitment to this forgiveness? Choose one to do today.

Consider this situation in which you are practising forgiveness. If it still feels hurtful, go through the inquiry steps again, and again . . . forgiveness is a constant act, an ongoing commitment.

26

BEING YOUR OWN WORST ENEMY

You are the most influential person in your life. What sort of companion do you want to be?

SPILT MILK

I'm tired today. I feel flat and down. I don't know if what I'm doing as a mum today is good or right. I'm overwhelmed by my feelings. I'm in a funk, and it feels like I'll never come out of it. I feel anxious, depressed, and down. I feel friendless.

I have to keep going, of course, and I will, of course. There are school lunches to make, a wash to hang out, an orthodontist to decide about, a school trip to pay for, a daughter with a playground politics hurt to be alongside.

I feel mechanical, one foot after the next. My joy feels so far away, my whoomph and verve like some kind of vanished summer holiday. I feel embarrassed to even feel like this—vulnerable about my flawed, pathetic self, so critical of myself that I'm not able to touch the joy of my being alive. When I feel good, I feel so able. This feels so disabling.

My eleven-year-old calls from school. She feels sick. Wants to come home. I hear myself: compassionate, understanding, supporting, checking, forgiving. "Oh, sweetheart, that's no good, sure, just come home. Do you feel like eating? I'll pick you up, no, I'm not mad at you, these things just happen . . ."

How come I don't do that for myself?

Instead, I hear a voice telling me, *Just get on with it. Grow up. Get over yourself. Stop overthinking. Stop overfeeling.*

Part of me wants to snuggle up in a blanket in a safe lap and cry. But I'm a mother and an adult. Blankets and laps aren't so readily available unless I'm providing them.

So how am I going to deal with myself? Can I be that caring and loving person for myself?

Being Your Own Best Friend

Meeting the internal challenges of motherhood can be very demanding. You won't always feel on top of things, or joyous, or content. But that is no reason to give up on yourself or the value of the journey.

There are ways of being with yourself that are friendly and ways that are not. If you are tormenting yourself with doubt and shame, it will not be comfortable being you. But believe it or not, there is learning here, too!

The practice here is being your own best friend. Today is the perfect time to practise compassion, friendliness, love, patience, and forgiveness with yourself, just as you would for your beloved child or dear friend. Today, that beloved child, that dear friend, is you. Shift your course just one degree of kindness now, and you'll end up in a completely different place.

Appreciate that you are learning. Value your journey as a mother. Your patience and love can benefit you also; they're not just for others. Feeling crap is nothing to be ashamed of. It is an opportunity to be kind to yourself. Remember, you are speaking to the divine energy that is manifest in your being as you. Speak to yourself as your own best friend, warm, compassionate, and loving.

"You are doing your best." "Let this day go; start afresh tomorrow." "Give yourself the hug you need right now." "C'mon, let's run you a warm bath." "How about you just put your legs up the wall for five minutes." "You have done enough for now." Soften into the challenges, the learning, and your journey.

BEING YOUR OWN BEST FRIEND: INQUIRY

Describe a recent moment where you were your own worst enemy and the thoughts and feelings that went with this.

As a compassionate, friendly, loving, patient friend, what would you say to someone who felt like this?

What could your ultimate best friend say and do for you right now?

Note two things you could do to **be your own best friend** and practise them both in the next twenty-four hours.

Note here what you did and the effect on you. What understanding are you gaining about **being your own best friend**?

27

GUILT, REGRET, HOPELESSNESS, AND DESPAIR

It's not what you did that matters; it's what you do next. How we respond to each moment moves us toward or away from living our lives as we want to.

SPILT MILK

Things are less than perfect. I've just snapped; I shouted at my children. I should be better at this by now. I am overwhelmed by mountains of washing, crying kids, low energy. And I still haven't been to the supermarket . . .

I am not gliding through motherhood. My kids are alive, loved, safe, well housed, well fed. I am a doting advocate for them in health and education, but I feel like I'm not handling the domestic, logistical, emotional, and psychological demands of motherhood so well. Thousands of challenges big and small are mounting up in my day. I get stressed, cycle around in frustration and resentment, spew it out, feel bad, and end up at despair. My purpose of staying steady and loving of myself and others feels like an impossibility. I feel guilty, hopeless, defeated.

I'm tired of trying to do better. I feel like I can't. No matter how hard I try, I can't shift the concrete block of doubt that sits in my chest. Anxiety, frustration, and uncertainty seem to be my life companions. I wonder if I'll ever be at peace, easy, steady, clear.

Am I like this because of my genetics? If I'm hardwired, there's nothing I can do; no amount of intention and willpower is going to shift my nature. If it's nurture, it's how I was raised. Are my parents to blame for my neuroses and deficiencies, their parents for theirs in turn? If so, my kids will be my hapless victims.

But as much as I feel like succumbing to moods and impulses, I do believe that through insight into my functioning and practising conscious responses, I can become wiser and more content. I do have a choice. So what shall I do in the face of this despair?

Focus on the Next Step

Tangled-up kids: *You made me do it. She hit me back first.* Tangled-up adults: *Oh, I shouldn't have done that. I'm so angry at myself. I've let myself down again . . .* caught in what went wrong and bad. Sound familiar?

Spilt milk tangles are only reinforced and further tangled by inquisitions of hurt, justifying "right" and "wrong" motives, and apportioning blame.

It happened. Your life is lived in what you do next.

If you feel guilty, regretful, hopeless, or despairing about something you've done, now is not the time to turn against yourself. Turn toward yourself instead. Giving yourself a hard time when you're already having one will trap you back there in the old. Rather than going over all the things you've done wrong, turn your attention to now. In these difficult moments, it is important to liberate yourself to act with intention and purpose.

The practice here is focus on the next step. It's not what you did that matters; it's what you do next. Free yourself to act now. Your next step determines what you create in your life.

Don't go back into the tangle. The tangle is tempting, but it will keep you in the past, and that is not where you'll create a new response. You can only change things by doing something new now. It might be hard, but it's a chance to break the old cycle.

This is not forgive and forget; it is forgive and let your next action liberate you. Update! Now! Take the next step consciously.

FOCUS ON THE NEXT STEP: INQUIRY

Describe a current or recent tangled or despairing mothering moment.

What thoughts, feelings, and actions hold you in the tangle?

Focus on the next step. What do you want to create in this new moment?

How could you do this?

Practise **focusing on your next step** in your mothering day today and note your discoveries here.

ANGER

*Fear and anger are telling you
something. Don't judge or punish
yourself, thinking, "I'm a bad
person." Go gently with yourself.
Listen for self-knowledge with
courage and care.*

SPILT MILK

I feel angry at my kids for dumping bags, shoes, and jackets in the hallway just after I cleaned and tidied the house. Another day, this may not bother me, so it's not the bags or my kids making me angry. It's me.

I feel unappreciated and unsupported. I feel bad that I feel like this.

How do I express my anger as a mother? Do I protect my kids from it, pretend it isn't there, and fake external calm while gritting my teeth till they crack? Do I give in to the pull of emotion over reason, have a tantrum, let the world know how I feel so I can get it off my chest and move on? I have shouted, cried, blamed, fumed, and seethed. I have dropped to the floor to stop myself exploding outwards. I have jumped up and down until the anger spell broke and then laughed at the ridiculousness of my tangled reasoning.

I explode and throw the washing basket. *CRASH!* I see my little one's tear-welled face shocked by the outburst from the scary beast that was mummy and hear her ask, "When is Daddy coming home?" I feel horrible. I never want my children to be scared of me.

"Why?" my fifteen-year-old texts when I ask for her sleepover address and landline. I'm outraged. I said "Yes" to her, and she says "No" to me. It's not reciprocal. I feel restrictive and untrusting, threaten instant collection, lecture about responsibility, trustworthiness, and safety. She wants independence. I want reliable connection, for her safety and for my peace of mind. It is reasonable to ask. I feel furious at her belligerent ignorance.

When I calm down enough to listen to my anger, it helps me get clear. *This is not okay by me, and that is enough of a reason!* These are my terms: no address, no sleepover. It is a relief to be so clear.

Listening to Anger

Anger is an indicator that things are not okay for you in your world. Anger may come from feeling hurt or powerless and can be triggered suddenly in reaction to old cues. Irritation, annoyance, disappointment, resentment, shock, frustration, and anxiety are all early warning messages. Who is sending you these messages? YOU are! It is important that you pay attention.

Motherhood will give you plenty of opportunities to meet your anger. You may feel angry when your kids don't do what you tell them to when you tell them, angry at housework, angry that you're not in control, even angry that you're angry! From feeling tense to a surging stomach, from seeing red to blind rage, anger has a powerful physical effect on the body. As an emotion, anger can feel so inside you, so visceral, but it is not you.

Anger is where you'll get stuck unless you learn to read the signs.

If you can know the point of your anger, there is a way to work with it and to have it work for you. Look to where the signpost is pointing, not at the sign. Back there at the origin fifteen minutes ago, or fifteen years ago, something has snagged you. Slow down; apply your consciousness. Ask: *What is the reason for my anger? What do I need?*

The practice here is listening to anger. By listening to anger and what is behind it, you can gather insight into your functioning. From here, you can choose to act in ways that honour you and the situation.

What you learn from your anger could liberate you!

LISTENING TO ANGER:
INQUIRY

Recall a recent mothering moment when you felt angry, and describe how you responded.

Finish these sentences:
I felt angry because . . .

Behind my anger is the feeling of/idea that/worry of/fear that . . .

What response is left over in you now?

Listen to your anger. What message are you sending yourself?

What response to this message would honour yourself and the situation?

How could you carry **listening to anger** into your mothering day?

29

MY ANGER
HABIT

*In moments of anger, we
need to take care—care of
ourselves, care of others, care
of our anger; we need to take
the care we are longing for.*

SPILT MILK

Mornings are becoming a nightmare. Why won't my family just do what I ask when I ask and GET READY? My getting-everyone-ready-in-the-morning stress is no fun; not for me, my kids, my husband; not for anyone. I feel stuck, angry, at a loss as to how to shift this pattern. Mornings just won't go away!

There has to be a better way. My husband and I make a plan: at flash o'clock tomorrow morning, I will go for a walk up the hill behind our house. It will have the joint effect of getting me out of the house, out of everyone's faces, them out of mine, and me out of feeling ensnared in habitual frustration and anger, and I'll get some much-needed exercise. And okay, I confess, I figure *he'll* have to do my job and find out how hard it is.

I fume my way up the hill. I puff. I look at the sky. I smell the grass. I start to feel lighter. This is a much better option!

Then I worry. What is happening at home . . . what will I find when I get back?

I can barely recall now what I found, but whatever it was it didn't have my stuck frustration at the helm. I went again, kept going. Sometimes I returned to partial chaos, sometimes to proud self-organization. It didn't matter. After time on my own to breathe and reflect, I was more able to accept whatever was happening.

Years later, my morning run has become a valuable habit in my life. I run a hill track at dawn with a friend. It sets me up much better to meet the challenges of my day.

In fact, if I don't run for a couple of days and I'm getting irritable, my kids say, "Mum, have you had your run today?"

Taking Care of Anger

Are you dismayed and surprised when anger shows up? If anger is a regular caller, accept its certain visit and plan in advance. Recognising your anger habits allows you to anticipate getting angry and prepare yourself to vent safely before or when you are in the heat of it. Getting familiar with your anger enables you to direct your anger, instead of the other way around.

The practice here is taking care of anger. Taking care of anger may sound like an astonishing approach, but if you are feeling injustice, stress, hurt, or fear, you do not need a fight with yourself; you need care and consideration. Below are some ideas for safe venting strategies in the heat of the moment from small to big.

- Recognise it: Know your habits. *I often feel irritable when I'm parking my car/at this time of day/when I'm vacuuming.*
- Name it early: *I feel ratty./This feeling is anger.*
- Steady it: Take five deep, slow, diaphragm-swelling breaths.
- Embrace it: Go into "child's pose"/relax your body/feel your breath/cry/ask for a hug/hug yourself/breathe.
- Express it: Rather than hurtful words, let out the sound *Roaaar!*/Shout "I'm feeling angry!"
- Move it: Leave the room/pull the car over and get out/ dance/tense and release your muscles.
- Exhaust it: Take it out on a pillow or bean bag/have a jumping tanty to use your adrenaline/do ten Sun Salutes/get out of the house and run the block.
- In an emergency, if you are about to hurt yourself or someone else, drop to the floor.

New habits take practice. Be patient and forgiving while you learn to do something a new way.

TAKING CARE OF ANGER: INQUIRY

What do you habitually do when you are beginning to get angry?

What care do you want taken of you at these moments?

Write a list of new options for **taking care of anger** while it is small.

What do you habitually do when you are very angry?

What care do you want taken of you in these moments?

Write a list of new options for **taking care of anger** when it gets big.

What could you do to prepare for these new options?

If you think you need professional support, seek it and know that you are not alone. Motherhood profoundly challenges our deepest and oldest human behaviours. You have a potent opportunity for insight and change. Take the care you deserve.

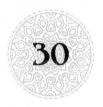

30

LOSING IT:
THE FIRE OF
MOTHERHOOD

*Did you "just lose it"? What
did you lose, your bad old
temper? Or did you lose your
intention, your purpose, your
sense of freedom to act from
love, joy, and appreciation?*

SPILT MILK

I'm trying to get everyone out of the house for school and work and LIFE. I'm trying to get my kids to behave in front of critical grandparents. I'm feeling pressured, tired, unsupported. I'm just holding on.

Things are mounting up, mounting up, until that one last straw, a ridiculously little thing, tips me over the edge of my managing strategies, past the point of no return. I snap, I surge, I stop holding it in, and I relinquish my sense of responsibility for that small moment of relief. I shout; I say something hurtful. I bash the red plastic fire helmet repeatedly on the edge of the dress-up trunk because "I JUST TIDIED UP THIS ROOM AND NOW LOOK AT IT!" I surrender to the release of roaring "JUST GET READY!!!!!!", to the fleeting satisfaction in snapping the toy that's causing the fight. THERE, that'll fix it!

But the satisfaction of reaction, the relief of not holding on any longer, is short lived. The instant I can think again and assess my mothering choice, the efficacy of my action looks ridiculous. Immediately, there's another choice: what to do next with what I've done? Guilt, shame, defensiveness, self-righteousness, depression, self-pity, or getting some better options. Now.

Apology. "Sorry; I didn't do that so well, did I! That wasn't my best option. I need help here."

I identify what started it. I'm trying to practise immediately what I could do differently next time. I welcome the Fire of Motherhood to burn that dross up, because it's got to feel better than this. If others are now angry or upset, I have to accept and work with that, too.

I want to learn from this.

Reading the Early Warning Signs

Have you ever said "I just lost it," "I just snapped," "I just exploded," or something similar? Most likely, you've been sending yourself messages and ignoring them. **The practice here is reading the early warning signs.** Tension builds in the body and mind like steam in a geyser. Little annoyances and anxieties accumulate and the pressure mounts up until "PSSHFFFT!"—big eruption, mud, ash, third-degree burns, and another big spilt-milk mess to clean up.

If you start the day with a negative thought—*I'm so tired, I'm not going to make it through the day*—you may already be at a 2 on the tension scale. A child resists going to school, you worry and go up to a 3. You feel irritation that the dishes weren't done last night, 4. To start breakfast means clearing yesterday's mess first, 5. "Someone ELSE please feed the cat," 6. "I said put your shoes on and brush your teeth!"—7. "STOP squabbling, you two!"—8. From here, you are past the TURN BACK signs, over the KEEP OUT barrier, and well into the DANGER zone. "Where are the keys?!"—9. You are just leaking gas for that one small spark . . . "Muuuum, I don't like hard eggs . . ." **BOOM!**

It's not that you just suddenly lost it when your seven-year-old complained about hard eggs; you began losing your way back at 4. If you recognise the early warning signs at a 4, you have more choice to take action and defuse your accumulating tension. It is easier to take action at 3 or 4. After 7, it is very difficult to turn back down the tension scale. At 4, you can still listen and take care of yourself, your concerns, and everyone around you. It takes effort, but you can turn it around.

READING THE EARLY
WARNING SIGNS: INQUIRY

Notice where you are on the tension scale right now (1 = relaxed, 10 = exploding). Describe what being at this number is like for you. What's happening in your body and mind?

Note what has occurred in your day to get to this point, what number you started your day at, and what took you up or down the tension scale.

Write down some strategies you could use between 4 and 7.

Today, simply notice through the day as you go up and down the tension scale, and mentally give yourself a number. Over the next week, use the tension scale as a reference, practice **reading the early warning signs** and use your strategies for coming down the tension scale. Note any discoveries here.

31

WHOSE ANGER
IS THIS?

*Knowing the difference between
your anger and someone else's
allows you stand on the solid
ground of your conscious intention
rather than jumping into the
quagmire of someone else's
emotions. It is of no use to either
of you to both drown in the bog.*

SPILT MILK

As a child, when I got angry, I was met with bigger anger in response to mine. It was as if I had no right to be angry and the bigger anger was out to overpower mine. It didn't take much for my anger to spark a bigger, more dangerous reaction that could throw the whole teetering family system into chaos. Not a good position to be in when you're small. Consequently, my anger got very tangled up with other people's anger. It became very hard to figure my way through my anger, from understanding what had caused it toward discovery and self-responsibility.

I have been practising steadfastness when my daughter rages so I don't get caught up in her anger. I stay very still and calm. I focus on my breath. I don't go into battle with her. This way, she has only to battle herself—to come to know her rage without the interference of mine. She rages externally and internally, and eventually, the storm blows itself out. When it does, there is only her debris to deal with, not mine as well; only she is responsible for anything broken. When she feels her need for connection, she can find me exactly where she left me. I haven't moved physically or been emotionally derailed by her anger. The reconnection, the apology, or the acknowledgement of the underlying hurt is clear. I can see her making the return trip to connection, understanding, and responsibility faster.

Thankfully, I don't have to deal with the guilty mess of unpicking my entangled reaction. I am clear and present for her when she returns. After all, fighting her hurt with my desire to overrule her anger hasn't worked yet.

I am loving the feeling of my own steadfastness arising, even under fire.

Steadfastness

Your anger is a powerful force. Other people's anger is a very powerful force too. Feelings of fear, fury, shock, or shame can flare up in immediate response to other people's anger. You may want to defend yourself, to fight back and overpower their anger, or to reject their anger as wrong.

Others may want to aggravate you so they are not alone with their feelings, or so they have someone else to blame. There are as many hooks in someone else's anger as are in yours!

The practice here is steadfastness. Stand steady on the solid ground of your own conscious intent. The angry brain is an emotional brain; it is in survival function and cannot reason. Very rarely do wise actions come in retaliation or anger. You have to hold fast, and stay conscious and steady in response to others' anger. Be the rock, not the storm.

Practise noticing other people's anger as separate from you.

I see you are feeling hurt.

I hear you are frustrated.

I sense your irritation.

I see your anger.

Then name your steadfast practice alongside their anger.

I am practising being with you as you are.

I am practising valuing your experience without fixing it for you.

I am practising steadying my breathing.

I am practising noticing that your anger is not mine.

STEADFASTNESS: INQUIRY

Recall a recent moment where someone around you got angry. Describe how that was for you.

What do you think was behind their anger?

What did you do in response?

What does being steadfast mean to you?

What are three things you could do to stay steadfast around other people's anger?

When you meet someone else's anger, practise steadfastness in your intention, and note your experience here.

PART FOUR

Shaucha

PURITY OF BEING

32

BUSHWHACKING, GARBAGE, AND MEDITATION

Not free for a ten-day retreat?
How about a ten-minute retreat
once a day, or a ten-breath
retreat every hour?

SPILT MILK

I know meditation is good for me. I *want* to meditate. I *want* the goodness. I have diverted, procrastinated, excused, and defaulted enough. Today, I commit to meditating every day this week.

Day one: Meditation is like bushwhacking. I stop, but my mind rushes on. I spend fraught minutes climbing through mental creepers, snagging on emotional vines, and pushing along through the thick undergrowth of distractions. I imagine thick bracken where a path once was, now overgrown. I'm trying to focus on my breath, trying to remember to say the mantra, trying not to think about all the things I am trying not to think about. Annoying mental commentary newscasts what I am seeing, feeling, thinking. Meditation is hard work. Where is the bliss and depth?

"Day one of a retreat is always garbage day for me," a friend says. It helps to know it's not just me. So I persist. Through the week, the image of the overgrown path repeats. I continue to bushwhack my way through meditation. Until unexpectedly, I emerge out of the bush at the edge of a huge, still lake; my deepest, stillest self. My reservoir. I stop bushwhacking, stop trying, stop everything, and just absorb the bliss of this place. Ahhh. I'm here.

Next, when I sit for meditation, I see a rough-hacked path. I follow it back to the lake of bliss. It's still there! Next time, the path is a little more trampled and open. The more I use the path, the easier it is to find my way back to that place of deep stillness.

It is so much easier to persist now. Some days are just track maintenance, but still I feel recharged, uplifted, and sustained.

One-Minute Meditation

I t is hard to connect to your inner peace when you are in the habit of rushing. But what if it took only one minute? Even one minute of meditation can make a big difference in your mothering day. Meditation makes inner space and calms the nervous system.

The practice here is one-minute meditation. Take one minute of the many in your day to stop doing and just be. By turning your focus inward, you can reconnect to your reservoir of inner peace.

It is better to develop a habit of one-minute meditations than random fifty-minute marathons. If getting to meditation is your biggest hurdle, committing to one minute is a great way to trick your resistance. *It'll be only one minute. I'll just grab one minute now.* You don't have to pressure yourself with finding and sticking to a one-hour slot. Aiming for a manageable one minute means you are more likely to succeed. And once you are sitting relaxed, focused on just being, you will find you sit for longer. One minute easily becomes five; five easily becomes ten.

Once you are there, sitting, you can just be. You may get interrupted; mothers do, often. Just make a start and do whatever time allows. You can come back to it. There will be more one-minute opportunities in your day, and every minute is valuable.

Adapt this to suit your mothering day. Try one-minute meditation while nursing your baby, sitting by while your child goes to sleep, with eyes open focused on a single point, while you continue with your mothering day. The amount doesn't matter; just do it.

ONE-MINUTE MEDITATION: INQUIRY

Describe how you are feeling now.

Take one minute to meditate now. Take a comfortable position with your spine upright but relaxed. Sit on a cushion on the floor in a comfortable cross-legged position or sit on a chair with your feet flat on the floor. Use cushions under your feet or knees if you need to. Place your hands on your knees or thighs, palms down. Close your eyes. Bring your attention to your breath. Take three conscious breaths; breathe all the way out slowly, allow your lungs to gently refill, then let your breath find its natural rhythm. On the out breath, let tension leave your body. Feel your shoulders and stomach relax to make an easy space for your breath. Relax your eyes, jaw, tongue, and mind. If you notice your mind getting caught up in thoughts, simply say to yourself, *Thinking*, and gently bring your mind back to focus once again on the breath. When you are ready, gently open your eyes.

Describe how you are feeling now.

Note anything else alive in you after this practice.

How or when could you use **one-minute meditation** to benefit your mothering day?

33

TELL-TALE
BREATHING SIGNS

*Breathing keeps you alive. Your
first and last breath are as
significant as every breath
in between.*

SPILT MILK

I catch myself holding my breath. I didn't even realise I was doing it! As I take a deep breath, I notice my jaw is set, my shoulders hunched. I breathe, stretch my jaw, slowly lower my shoulders. As I relax and breathe, I become aware of an anxiety and tension I have been holding unconsciously. It crawls down to my gut.

Later, waiting in the car, I notice I am holding my breath again. I slowly breathe, release shoulders, neck, jaw. I can feel my stomach, too, snaking with anxiety. As soon as I breathe, the feeling shifts. I experience relief. So why am I doing that? I've caught myself doing something habitual. Perhaps I can learn from this.

I tense up again to investigate, this time consciously. I hold my breath, clench my jaw, and tense my shoulders. It's as if I am braced against life's next moment. I feel worried. About being late for an arrangement I've made. I feel ready to defend myself, fight, resist. I feel fear and uncertainty at what might happen next. I am anticipating judgement. I hear the thoughts: *I'll be blamed. I'll get in trouble. I will be judged as incompetent and irresponsible.* Wow. The thoughts are pervasive and insidious. I am catastrophizing, living in a fearful prediction of the future. I'm trying to keep everyone happy. I have been holding my breath to try to prevent others being upset with me.

I let go, relax my body, and breathe mindfully. I notice where I am. I sit for a moment. *I am breathing in . . . I am breathing out. I am here now.*

I will make a call soon and let folks know I won't be rushing on the road and might be late. But for now, I just breathe. I am in this moment. Let the next moment come.

Mindful Breath

Do you sigh a lot, find yourself taking shallow, panicky breaths or even holding your breath? You may not even notice how you are breathing.

How you breathe affects your thoughts, and conversely, your thoughts affect your breath. If you take short, panicky breaths, you are likely to feel panicky. Scary thoughts and feelings will tighten your breathing. Your breath connects directly to your state of mind. Calming your breath will calm your mind.

The practice here is mindful breath. Turning your mind to the quality of your breath is a fundamental practice of yoga and meditation. Mindful breath is easily available as a practice because you're already breathing every moment of your day. You may not get to your yoga mat or to sit for meditation, but to breathe mindfully makes a yoga practice of the many mental postures you go through in your mothering day.

Mindful breath can bring self-knowledge. Bring your attention to your breath. Without altering it, simply notice it. If you catch a moment of disturbed breathing, maintain that pattern while you investigate the thoughts, feelings, and causes beneath it.

Mindful breath is a wonderful tool for resetting your equilibrium and coming back to yourself. Breathe out long three times, emptying your lungs, using your diaphragm. Then relax and let your breath come in through your nose, letting your lungs fill naturally. Let your shoulders relax, then your jaw, your brow. Breathe naturally.

Mindful breath assists you moving through your day connected to your centre, aware, calm, and at ease moment to moment.

MINDFUL BREATH: INQUIRY

When do you usually notice your breathing through your mothering day, and what do you notice?

Twice today, practise **mindful breath** toward:

1. Self-knowledge: Notice your breath. Follow the thoughts behind the quality of breathing. Do not judge your thoughts; just follow them. Note them here as specifically as you can, using full sentences, and see what you discover.

2. Resetting your equilibrium: Notice your disturbed state. Take three reset breaths, then breathe easily. What do you notice?

When might **mindful breath** assist you in your mothering day?

34

OLD LABELS AND
NASTY THOUGHTS

*How do you talk to yourself?
With words of scornful criticism
or with words of love and
encouragement? Words shape
thoughts and beliefs; be aware of
what you say.*

SPILT MILK

In my family of origin, we acquired labels. They may have been briefly relevant, but they stuck long term. I became the one who "never does the dishes." Of course, as an adult and mother running a household, doing a steady stream of dishes on a daily basis, this is a ridiculous label to apply to me now. Nonetheless, when my family gets together, out come the linty old labels, prejudices, and habitual phrases. I feel how it obstructs recognition of growth. Old labels need questioning, and restrictive family pictures need updating. I'm on the lookout as a mother as a new generation of labels is born.

Today: I am feeling so joyous! *Life is wonderful!* I think. *I feel so blessed.* Then I hear the counterthought: *Oh, but if something terrible happened to your husband or one of your children, you wouldn't feel like this.* Instantly, I feel doubtful and mistrusting of my joy. I am shocked at how I undermine my own joyfulness. It's like a warning: *Don't get too comfortable! Get ready for inevitable pain.* Where does this insidious scepticism come from? Do I think joy is naïve, delusional, unsustainable? It is time to review the beliefs I am living from!

Today: I catch myself reinforcing my belief that I don't have enough time by continually saying "I don't have enough time."

My youngest daughter has a short fuse at the moment. I say "at the moment" because I seem to remember that my oldest daughter had a short fuse some years back. I am using "at the moment" to unhook her, and me, from an assumption that she is her behaviour, long term. We change and develop. I want to see her afresh today, unfolding. Can I do that for myself also? Can I update my picture of myself to notice what is evolving and shifting?

Conscious Language

Language is a powerful shaper of experience. Underneath the language you use are inherent beliefs about yourself and the world. How you talk to yourself and your children about yourself, about them, and about the world has a profound effect.

Old and unhelpful phrases you made up, or that you heard someone else say about you a long time ago, may have snuck in and be whispering constantly or lurking in wait for their cue. *I'll never get this right. I can't sing. You've always had a hot temper. He never cooks. Shut up before you embarrass yourself.* These old sentences may even have been intended to protect you but resulted in generating fear and restriction. Old verdicts may be outright falsehoods but still have a powerful effect if they are the reference points you use to describe and direct your life.

The practice here is conscious language. Conscious language use is a discipline. Catching moments of negative and prescriptive language can be very tricky, especially when they are so insidious. Being alive to what you say to yourself and others is to be alive to intention and effect.

Is what you say congruent with your experience and values? Notice how you talk to yourself and in what tone; what you say about yourself to others; how you talk to, and about, your partner and children. Are the things you say accurate? Are they enabling or obstructing the behaviours and beliefs you want to cultivate?

You're trying your best; new skills take practice.

I have the time I have.

I'm not sure what to do, but I will figure something out.

CONSCIOUS LANGUAGE: INQUIRY

What qualities are you seeking to cultivate in your life as a mother currently?

Write out any habitual comments you use as a mother that support you in this.

What thoughts are behind these?

Write out any habitual comments or thoughts you use as a mother that obstruct you in this.

Take one and rephrase it in a way that cultivates the qualities of life you are seeking.

What would you like to carry from this **conscious language** practice into your mothering day today?

35

THAT'S RUINED
MY WHOLE DAY!

*What is the story you tell
yourself about your life?
Is it a tale of hardship
and pity, or of insight and
appreciation? What does the
story you tell awaken in you?*

SPILT MILK

I'm in the thick of the preschool years. From time to time, my sister, who has two older boys, phones to ask how I am doing. My answers vary wildly from day to day, from morning to afternoon, from hour to hour, even. Sometimes my day is going along fine and then . . . isn't, for any number of spilt milk reasons. Occasionally my day goes in the other direction from calamity to calm.

"How are you going?" she asks. *Generally? Or in the peak or trough of this moment?* I fear if I don't deliver full coverage, she'll get the wrong impression, either that I am desperate and struggling all the time or, even worse, just fine and needing no support! I try to catch the torrent of my day in a thimble of summary, but I'm at a loss as to how I really am going. How do I assess the range?

I tend to measure my day by the worst bit. In one spilt-milk moment, the buoyancy of the day's successes can ebb away, and I spend the rest of the day deflated and bruised. My whole day gets tarred by the distress of the pants-wetting disaster, the frustration of a missed appointment debacle, the emotional drain of refereeing a fairy-dress skirmish. I declare the entire day a write-off and limp on through to bedtime.

"As a mother, I prefer to think of it in half days," my sister tells me. Now there's an idea! Instantly, I can say, "It's been a good half day!" or, "Oh, well, we got to eleven a.m. and things went sideways, but that was just the morning. At midday, we just started again, and the afternoon has been great!"

What a difference! What a framework for forgiveness and success! With two half days, I can double my chances of having a good day right there.

AND NOW . . . Refreshing the Page

Things may have gone wrong in one part of your day, but it doesn't mean your whole life has to go wrong. Each moment is an opportunity to start afresh. Carrying a sense of resentment, regret, or hopelessness through your day is one response to spilt milk, and starting again with a sense of refreshed opportunity for the new is another.

This practice is refreshing the page. Let go the lingering story of what happened and start the next page now. If there is something challenging in your mothering day that you want to address, that is good to be aware of. Refreshing the page is not about forgetting; it is about waking up to the joy available in every moment. You cannot be downtrodden in a tide of accumulative despondency when you refresh the page of the present.

Yes, that may have been difficult grocery shopping with two hungry toddlers and a squalling baby, coaching a belligerent teenager to engage with household responsibilities, being up and down all night with an ill child while you suffered symptoms of your own, or missing an important appointment in the melee of mothering demands. Yes, these things are demanding. There may be systemic frustrations you want to remedy there. However, before you adjust the world or give up, here are two words of liberation for you to practise: AND NOW . . .

AND NOW is a new moment, a new hour, a new half day. AND NOW is an opportunity to refresh the page. That other stuff has happened already; it is not your entire life. AND NOW a new chapter begins. You are the author of your purpose.

AND NOW. . . REFRESHING
THE PAGE: INQUIRY

How are you going? Make an assessment of your mothering day so far.

What old story is lingering in you from an earlier time?

Note if there is anything unresolved you want to attend to.

What could you let go of by **refreshing the page** that would liberate you from the old story?

AND NOW? What do you want to cultivate going forward?

AND NOW how will you do this on the refreshed page of your mothering day?

36

PRACTISING HABITS IS A HARD HABIT TO PRACTISE

Practice means to do something over and over. To cultivate your practice habit, all you need to do is practice.

SPILT MILK

Today: I sit to meditate and find myself thinking about all the things I have to do. I have a habit of feeling overwhelmed. I heap on the demands. I get more overwhelmed. My habitual response to overwhelm is to try harder. I try being in the present. I try remembering to breathe. I try remembering the quote I'm contemplating. I try to let that go and change my state. I try. I try. I keep trying.

I need a new habit here. What is the opposite of overwhelm and trying? Acceptance! What if I practise acceptance? Today, I accept that my meditation is practice at being present in my day as an overwhelmed mother.

Today: When I sit to meditate, I choose to practise acceptance. I will unload my boat of expectations and practise accepting what comes. Soon I get distracted thinking about something I have to do, then I get distracted from my distraction, then I realise I am drifting. *Uh oh, I'm drifting—this isn't meditation!* But I'm practising acceptance. I go with accepting the drifting and manage to stay afloat for about fifteen minutes. It feels good. Very, very good. It's taken me a while to get here. It is like fitness; I have to practise to make progress. That fifteen minutes was so worth it.

Today: I've got only five minutes. Is it enough? Should I wait until I have a clear twenty minutes to sit? Or perhaps I should do something useful with my time . . . postponement is another habit! Habitually, I often try to squeeze in a few tasks before I sit for meditation then miss the opportunity. I have to be firm with myself in a new habit of prioritizing "just doing it." So today, I just do it, and I think, *This is so wonderful. WHY did I delay?*

Choosing Your Habits

More than circumstance, your thoughts and habits create your inner state. What thoughts and habits are shaping your experience? If you habitually rush, feel agitated, anxious, and overwhelmed, or catastrophize with thoughts of doom and defeat, then this will shape your experience of motherhood.

The practice here is choosing your habits. Choosing habits that free you from stress and cultivate peace can be only beneficial to you and your loved ones. What are you prepared to do to feel more peace, love, joy, and steadiness? Probably quite a lot, right?

What fosters your joy, encourages calm, acceptance, and appreciation? Choose a habit that will uplift your being. Be specific about what habit you want to grow, how you will practise it, and when. *To make a habit of gratitude, I will say grace with my family each night before we eat.* Repetition creates habits, so start small and user friendly with achievable goals that fit easily into your mothering day. *To create a habit of inner calm, I will set my phone reminder to practise ten mindful breaths every hour.*

Now amongst the busyness, when your four-year-old emerges enthusiastically from the bathroom clutching the empty toothpaste tube, shouting, "The toothpaste is really long!", you are more able to respond from the inner calm you are cultivating.

If old habits, like impatience and defeat, get in your way when practising a new habit, you can turn them around. Impatience is unpractised patience; defeat is unpractised success. What do you need to do to practise patience or success?

CHOOSING YOUR HABITS: INQUIRY

What habits of thought and action connect you to your joy and intention as a mother?

What habits of thought and action disrupt your joy and intention as a mother?

Choose one quality you are wanting to cultivate in your life.

What habit could you practise to assist this? Be specific about when, where, and how.

What is likely to enable and hinder you in practising this new habit?

What could you set up for yourself to support yourself cultivating this habit?

Use the habit-forming chart at the back of this book to help you.

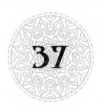

I DON'T HAVE ENOUGH TIME!

This is the time you have.
There is no other time.
Time is not waiting for you
somewhere else.

SPILT MILK

Today: I decide to use my meditation time to sort my office and to meditate in the evening. Not a good idea. I miss my recharge in the day. I do meditate, but it is late and I am tired.

Today: I sit as soon as I put baby down for her sleep, when I am not too tired. This is the time! Now! When time is on my side and I can meditate for as long as I need. It's better when my meditation determines the time I sit for, not the time I have determining the length of my meditation. When I do meditate, it is beautiful—I feel it strongly in my heart. It is bliss!!

Today: There is not enough time. I am rushing all morning, and the things TO DO are mounting up. I'm doing well so far, but it's pressured. It doesn't feel good. I'm chanting in my head, *Come on, come on, come on . . .* I get the kids up, breakfasted, dressed, hair brushed, wash on, bags packed, rabbits fed, kitchen tidied, beds made, lunches made, myself showered and dressed, wash out, 3x teeth brushed, prepared for work, organised, out the door, walk the kids to school, get myself to work . . . I am harried, irritated, pushing, rushing against the clock.

My kids don't move fast enough when I want them to; they dawdle, drift, distract, and detonate. It's not just a case of ticking a simple activity off a list. "Hair brushed" or "kids dressed" sounds simple, but it may just be the title of a full-scale Peking opera.

What contortions I put myself through to shepherd my kids through the schedule of the day! All the while, I have a persistent sense that I'm behind. So much rests on getting things done in time. Anxiety increases; joy decreases.

Making Friends with Time

As mothers, there is an inevitable need to do many things at once. These things may be important and necessary, but if your solution is going faster and doing more, what suffers ultimately is you, a mother in hyperdrive trying to do it all. You may live in an anxious future of never-ending TO DO tasks, or run behind trying to catch up to past expectations, but you will not be here, now.

Is your relationship to time serving your purpose? Are you allowing yourself to appreciate the time you have and what you do with it? Or are you squeezing yourself, your children, and your adrenal glands into an overstuffed schedule? Why? Do you think satisfaction will come only after you've "done it all"?

There is another way to be that is less hectic and creates more joy and love as you go. Rather than making yourself a victim of time, can you get time on your side? If you find yourself blaming time, wishing for more time, or pushing against time, finding a friendlier way to work with time will connect you to yourself and your deepest intention.

The practice here is making friends with time. You have the time you have. There is no point wishing you could have been more spacious, more loving and playful as a mother once your kids leave home. Today is the time to be the mother you want to be. Rather than approaching time resentfully and complaining that it's not enough, value time as your friend, abundant and generous, allowing you to do what is important to you. Everything takes time, and in return, time gives opportunity. Take the time needed to cook dinner spaciously, to cut your child's nails lovingly, to get across town to four p.m. karate easefully. Be real about the time each task deserves as an act of love and joy.

MAKING FRIENDS WITH TIME: INQUIRY

What are you wanting to cultivate in the mothering day ahead of you?

How could your relationship with time support this?

Write a list of things you intend to do in your mothering day today.

Note next to each thing:

- how much time you allow in your mind for this thing
- how much time each thing is *actually likely to take*
- the inner state you want to experience while doing this task

Choose one of the TO DO tasks from your list. What might prevent you experiencing this state while you carry out this task?

What would support your experiencing this inner state while you carry out this task?

Practise **making friends with time** today and note any discoveries here.

38

COMPARISON

*If you find yourself
comparing yourself to others,
come back to your breath.
Where there is breath, there
is life. Where there is life,
there is creativity. You have
the gift of life. Start with
that. The inner self has no
need for comparison.*

SPILT MILK

I compare myself to others: my life, my mothering, my house, my choices, my everything. It's a habit that has me gazing over the fence at someone else's grass and seeing it as greener.

My husband takes the kids Saturday-morning grocery shopping while I stay home to clean the house. I am angrily vacuuming; I am furiously cleaning the bathroom. I am getting the big list of jobs done, quickly cramming as much in as I can before they get home.

The estimated return time passes. I keep cleaning. Eventually, they arrive home. They've had a great time, shopped and bought pastries, then stopped at the park on the waterfront; he's had a beer and mussels while the kids ate fries and played nearby. How irresponsible! How annoying!

"Right!" I say. "Next time, I do the fun job and you stay home!"

So next Saturday, I take the kids shopping; I get the job done, we stop at the park. It is cold. The good time eludes me. We go home.

Ha! I think. *How's he going with the crap job?* Guess what? Music is playing, incense is wafting through the house, the house is cleaner and tidier, and he's had a great morning.

I thought the grass was greener in this paddock, but now that I'm in it, the paddock I was in before looks better. It's comparison. Oh, I get it. This is my life, my paddock, my grass. I choose what crop I plant and what fertiliser I use.

Rather than gazing comparatively over the fence at someone else's grass, I need to be more purposeful with my own paddock, choose what I grow and reap, find the joy available in my own green grass, get off what others are doing, and focus on creating my own good time.

Living with Clear Purpose

Motherhood is rife with comparison: comparisons between pregnancies, births, children, their development, mothering styles, work choices, home life, schools, achievements, bodies, and more. Anxiously comparing yourself as "more" this, "less" that, or "better" or "worse" than someone else will leave you feeling fragmented, isolated, and alone. You may think others are mothering effortlessly while you struggle to get places on time, manage a library tantrum, or make choices about screen time and lunchbox food. Gliding through motherhood, or appearing to, in control and unscathed, is not the goal here. The truth is far richer than that. You have your own life to live, your own custom-made joys and troubles to meet and grow with. Judging yourself as superior or inferior to others distracts you from living your life and embracing its many unique lessons. So what keeps you on your track?

The practice here is living with clear purpose. Are you living life as you want to? When you live purposefully, according to your values, you will feel aligned, potent, and fulfilled. When you compromise your values, you will feel conflicted, frustrated, and powerless. Clarifying your values strengthens resolve, reduces internal conflict, and sets your journey by the compass of your own intention. When you are clear on your values, you will have purpose by which to guide your choices and actions. When you live in alignment with your heart, there is no need for comparison.

As a mother, you have an opportunity to know the breadth of your being, to learn life's richest lessons in love and acceptance, and to be your best, most loving self. Living with clear purpose gives value to every moment of your mothering journey.

LIVING WITH CLEAR PURPOSE: INQUIRY

List the five things most important to you about life. State what you mean and why it is important to you.

Score yourself out of 10 for how fully you are currently living these values. Note below why this is the score.

If you had a mission statement for your life, what might it be? *My purpose in life is to . . .*

If you had a mission statement in your life as a mother, what might it be? *My purpose as a mother is to . . .*

How will you enact **living with clear purpose** in the day ahead of you?

39

JUDGEMENT

*Discernment is a guide to
knowing what will move you
toward or away from yourself.*

SPILT MILK

As I go to my crying baby, my mother-in-law says, "We just used to leave our babies to cry." This might mean *I wish I'd been encouraged to follow my instincts and pick my baby up if I felt it was the right thing to do; I like the way you are mothering.* Maybe it's concern: *You're working too hard.* I'm sleep deprived and trying to figure out what to do and feeling very observed in my attempts and failings. I just feel defensive and unsupported. I feel like it's veiled criticism: *You are doing it wrong. You are indulging yourself and spoiling your child. I don't like the way you are mothering.* I'm doing my best, I'm learning, I don't know what is right, I'm just trying things out. I feel judged, inadequate, lonely. Nothing is built between us except distance.

I feel judgement through Christmas holiday with my wider family: about me, my mothering, and my children. My children's behaviours are a reflection of my failings: I haven't disciplined them enough, I'm doing it the wrong way, or I let them get away with too much. My father says, "You're a great mum . . . I didn't think you would be." I'm dumbfounded. Great—that I've proved him wrong in some previous conclusion he had of my perceived shortcomings. My sister says, "What a shame your youngest is copying her big sister's behaviour." I'm astonished. Some verdict has found my oldest daughter objectionable, and now my previously unblemished youngest is tarnished by her.

I know about this kind of judgement, because I do it too. Embroiled in petty machinations, I judge others' behaviours as proof of their fallibility and interpret the world in my favour.

What do I take on from others judgement? What is my responsibility with my own? Can I turn judgement to a purpose that builds connection, love and acceptance?

Discernment

Everyone is an expert on mothering because they've all got one. Many people are experts on mothering because they are mothers or are close to one. There are many forces at work on you as a mother: social, cultural, familial, historical, educational, economic, external, and internal. There are many ideas, expectations, and judgements about how, what, and who you should be as a mother. Judgement can condemn, undermine learning, and derail self-determination, or it can be used to connect you to your purpose. So how do you navigate expectation and judgement in a way that strengthens you and your purpose?

The practice here is discernment. Discernment is the process of "better judgement" by which you ascertain which things nourish and support your spirit and journey, and those that do not. Noting the effect people and situations have on you will assist you in knowing what to move toward and what to move away from. Discernment is the process of asking, *Does this situation support my peace and ease? Do I feel energised, affirmed, and loved when I spend time with this person?* If you feel uplifted, seen, loved, at ease, then this is something to move toward. If a person or situation leaves you feeling doubtful, inferior, depleted, or undermined, then it is not supporting you in your journey.

If a close person or situation is causing you distress, discernment will assist you in deciding what next step to take. Ask yourself: *What do I want to grow in my life? What next step shall I take with this situation?* Discernment will guide you toward your own wisdom, joy, and purpose. And when judging others, the same questions apply.

DISCERNMENT: INQUIRY

What things, people, places, and situations uplift and sustain you in your journey through motherhood? Be specific.

What is strengthened in you by these things?

What things or people undermine and drain you in your journey through motherhood?

What is one quality you want to experience more of in your life?

How might you use **discernment** to grow this in the week ahead?

How might you use **discernment** to grow this in your day today?

40

AM I A GOOD ENOUGH MOTHER AND YOGI?

*When we appreciate that
everything we do—all of
our responses, our choices,
our reflections—brings
us closer toward our goal,
then nothing, no choice, no
response, is wasted.*

SPILT MILK

I feel as if there's too much to do in the mothering duties of my daily life. With no uninterrupted time out for me, I can't unwind enough to be physically and mentally still. I feel held back from making progress in my inner life because I'm constantly feeling challenged and at the edge of my capacity. *I believe I can't do enough.*

Perhaps I'll have to wait until my kids are old enough before I can get back to myself, get my meditation practice going again, go on a retreat or two, make some really consolidated progress . . . but it's a long time to wait, and it's a very intense, noisy, busy, toy-strewn waiting room.

Perhaps I'm just not a good enough yogi, not dedicated enough to my practices and path.

Perhaps I'm not a good mother, not dedicated in the right ways and doing the right things. I remember reading about the concept of "The Good Enough Mother." D. W. Winnicott, who coined the concept, said the good enough mother is the best kind there is; in her "ordinary devotion," she meets her infant's needs, but in the context of the real world, she sometimes fails to. The child, while essentially held and safe, increasingly learns to meet the world. Phewf! I am a good enough mother!

Perhaps "ordinary devotion" could apply to being a "good enough yogi." Pursuing enlightenment in the real world of mothering, meeting the challenges and bumps of ordinary living. In my ordinary devotion, I meet my imperfections. That in itself is good enough; in fact, it's perfect!

I am a good enough yogi, practising ordinary devotion in the real world of mothering.

Being Good Enough

Meeting the demands of motherhood can feel like running on the spot in a dream, the monster close behind, your heart thumping and no sense of forward motion. If you are used to the expectations of a being a high-achieving, autonomous career woman or thrive on "getting the job done," the captive monotony of looking after little children can be incredibly challenging. With your own children, that feeling is intensified, because more than anything else, you'll want to do it really well, for them and for you.

How do you measure a sense of progress and worth in the detailed ordinariness of a humdrum mothering day? High expectations of yourself and slow, unmeasurable results are at odds with the sense of progress you may be used to. If you find a sense of progress in motherhood elusive, you'll need a new point of reference to measure the value of what you are doing.

The practice here is being good enough. Some days will feel good, and some will not; it doesn't mean progress is not being made or that you are not fulfilling your purpose. It is important to appreciate the discoveries and new understandings emerging and accumulating through your mothering days. Capturing them strengthens a sense of value in days that can otherwise feel very repetitive. If what you expect from your mothering day is unrealistic, you won't feel progress. If what you seek is aligned with living your values, you will have a mother-appropriate frame and know the value of being good enough.

What are your reference points for enough-ness? Do they support you in your journey? If you can't do enough, can you be enough?

BEING GOOD ENOUGH:
INQUIRY

What does your mothering day involve today?

What do you expect of yourself in this?

What would be good enough?

What does your life as a spiritual being involve today?

What do you expect of yourself in this?

What would be good enough?

Carry this frame of practising **being good enough** into your day, and note the effect here.

41

SELF-CENTRED, SELF-INDULGENT, SELFISH!

If you grapple with the idea that self-care is selfish, self-indulgent, or unnecessary, then ask yourself, "How am I going with this approach?"

SPILT MILK

I'm so knackered. I would have a lie down, but there's so much to do. I'd feel better if my bed was made, the hand basin clean, the dinner on, and the washing folded; if I used my daughters' sleep time to DO something useful.

I would have a meditation, but I can't sit still for the list of stuff inside my head. Rather than thinking about all the stuff I could be doing, why don't I just get on with it and cut out the time-wasting?

Rather than going to yoga, a movie, a walk, anything that isn't a necessary task, why don't I just . . . what? Do something else more productive, more valuable, more justifiable?

Somehow, looking after myself is so far down the list, I feel unable to, like it's not important. If I am not actively stretched somehow, it is proof that I am lazy, not trying hard enough, not deserving of the rewards that come from hard work, commitment, and sacrifice.

The rules in my head say, *Do everything before you rest!* But what if there is no end to the "everything" to be done? What if I'm exhausted? Where is the break? I am my own worst boss.

I need to wake up my inner "good boss." If my job was caring for myself, I'd say, "You're tired. Stop for now. You've done a great job! But now you need to rest. Figure it out in the morning when you've had a sleep. Don't pick up anything else. Just go to bed."

Why is that so hard? I feel if I don't soldier on, it is proof that I'm weak, selfish, self-indulgent, and lazy. But, surely, caring for myself *is* part of my job . . .?

Self-Care

Mothers look after others. Who looks after the mothers? Even with people in your life who care for you and love you, you need to take care of yourself. Biologically and emotionally, you need sleep and nourishing food. Obviously, the early years of motherhood are not the place to expect unbroken sleep, but where sleep is broken, it is wise to allow for that and top up with something restorative that replenishes you and acknowledges your need for rest.

The practice here is self-care. Self-care is identifying your own need and choosing something that nourishes you at your core, physically, emotionally, psychologically, and spiritually.

Self-care supports you in your journey. Some things will knock you off your perch, leave you depleted and less resourced; others assist you in staying steady and unfolding your joy more and more.

Read through the following and consider your relationship to each. *Exercise. Food. Meditation. Yoga. Sleep. Housework. Work. Asking for help. Paying for help. Time to yourself. Connection to others. Friends. Family. Social time. Relaxation. Sex. Intimacy. Affection. Caring for others. Being cared for.*

It is important to be centred in yourself. You are the foundation of your family. Let yourself have some of the mothering love you so readily give to your children.

Prioritizing acts of care for yourself as a mother will most certainly benefit you—and not only you!

SELF-CARE: INQUIRY

In what ways do you care for yourself as a mother?

In what ways do you not care for yourself as a mother?

What underlying thoughts do you have about self-care?

What ways would you like to care for yourself more?

Choose one. Picture it happening, and describe when, where, and how you could do this.

What things might stop you doing this act of self-care?

What are you wanting to grow in this act of self-care?

Undertake to practise this act of self-care. Report back here on how it went. If necessary, adapt and try again.

42

BIRTH AND SEX: WHAT HAPPENED TO MY BODY?

Your body followed an astonishing process of creation, a creativity as awe inspiring and wonderful as the formation of the universe. What a body you have! What a marvellous wonder! It is a thing to be celebrated, revered, and treasured.

SPILT MILK

My body dial has been on "Lover" setting for so many years. Now, abruptly, it's switched to "Mother." My breasts, my vagina, my everything has a new overriding function. And it's not only *my* body anymore; it's someone else's address, life support, and food source. My aching mammary glands swell to the size of watermelons until there's cleavage between my shoulder blades. I was never a buxom lass, so my husband can't believe the tantalizing transformation. "Touch these and you die," I say. I am sore, aching, sleep deprived, and excruciatingly sensitive. Any nipple stimulation and I switch automatically into mummy mode, with toe-curling letdown, spraying the room like a shower nozzle with fine threads of milk. It's not sexy for me at all. It's maternal.

My vagina is a new territory altogether, carrying sensitive tear scars, pouting elasticity. And my libido . . . well, I have another focus, and I'm too exhausted by bedtime for anything but sleep. I'm too exhausted any time of the day. I am all gived out. I have no room in my head for eroticism while I listen atavistically for my baby stirring. When my husband wants sex, it's one more request for my body to do something for someone else. I just want a sleep, a shoulder rub, a cuddle.

So it goes, until we have the talk. The talk starts something like "What are we going to do about our sex life?" We don't want this to be the end, so we have to get inventive, pay attention to what is new, take a new approach. It takes time, but we keep talking.

We start again, listening to this new body, this new us, new sensations, a new honesty, and discover to our delight a whole new world of intimacy, pleasure, and love. Some things just got even better!

Honour Your Body

Giving birth and becoming a mother changes your body. You have carried, swollen, grown an entirely new organ, hosted a hiccupping, fidgeting body inside yours, stretched, contracted, given birth with extreme chthonian messiness, vomit, blood, fluids, and faeces. You have lactated, breastfed, held, or known sensations particular to sharing your heart, body, and mental space in other ways. You have experienced the miracle of bringing another being into the world. You are a phoenix from the flames of birth, a woman who has travelled where no man can, no matter how many extreme sports he may use to test his limits.

The practice here is honour your body. This body you have is the temple in which you live, a creator of life; it deserves care and reverence. Purity of being is cultivated in the care you take of your sacred body, what you put into it, and how you think about it. Treat your body in ways that make you feel clear and connected to your divinity. Love your whole self as you are. Respect your body with good food, nourishing sleep, thoughts of appreciation, and gratitude for the marvellous body you have. Listen to the inner changes; celebrate the outer changes brought about by birth as markers of your miraculous life-giving journey.

Cultivating purity of being includes your relationship to your body, and this also includes sex. You are a mother, not a celibate monk. As a mother, you embody the human capacity for greater love, intimacy, insight, and connection to self, others, and the miracle of life. Pay attention to what honours your body and sense of self, and what doesn't. Listen to what sustains and uplifts you, to what builds stronger recognition of your divinity.

HONOUR YOUR BODY:
INQUIRY

What changes have occurred in your body through becoming a mother?

How do you feel about these changes?

What do you appreciate about your body through the process of becoming a mother?

Describe the relationship you would like to have with your changing body.

What things do you do that **honour your body**?

Name some ways you can further uplift and nurture your being through **honouring your body**.

PART FIVE

Ishvarapranidhana

ACKNOWLEDGING THE
SPIRITUAL NATURE
OF BEING

43

ANYWHERE BUT HERE

Welcome yourself to the present.

SPILT MILK

Today, I commit to an extended meditation. *Will I survive? Will I be too agitated? Will I get there?* I close my eyes.

I feel a pressure to meditate the "right" way. I'm finding sitting still really hard. I fidget, I sneeze, I need to blow my nose. My knees hurt. *Shall I just give up? Is it really doing me any good?* But I have committed!

I decide just to be curious. Inside me, I see a light, burning orange in the deep, dark redness. Spiralling downward, it moves like a flare, slowly descending. With a pulsing energy, I follow. Down it goes, curving clockwise to encircle my heart, then it continues its path down through my chest, slowly, coming to rest in the central point between my upper ribs, below my breastbone. This is the place I feel tight and sore when I am anxious and stressed.

In my head, there is an annoying voiceover of what is going on, a self-conscious description of my experiences as if I'm recounting it to someone later. I want to be present, so I put the commentary into the present tense. *I see a tunnel of light, and I am following it. It curves down and around, colour swirls, patterns pass, pulsing, repeating.* I move toward and away from the present.

Then, suddenly, I am looking at a luminous blue pool of light. I stay by it. Play with trying to get in it, be immersed in it. The commentary stops for a short time, and I am bobbing around in the present. I hear the thought, *Don't try to do anything. Don't fight your thoughts. Just be in the present.* This stays with me. I can sit, just sit. Even if I find trying to meditate too intense, I can just rest in this space, with my eyes closed, in the present.

Being Where You Are Right Now

Yoga is more than bending into poses that strengthen, discipline, and extend your body. It is also an attitude toward living and the engagement of practices that assist to strengthen, discipline, and extend your inner self. The very act of breathing itself becomes yoga if you turn your conscious awareness to it.

The practice here is being where you are right now. Turn your conscious awareness to what you are doing in each moment. So much time is spent anticipating the future or tangled in the past, it is easy to miss being where you are right now.

Mothers do many things again and again. If you are tired, rushing, or thinking about the next thing you will do after the thing you are doing now, you will miss the present. A meal can be cooked, a swing pushed, a slow meandering walk to the shop taken, a book read, teeth brushed, and an entire day lived on autopilot.

Each moment of the day is different from the last and worthy of note. It is a practice to keep refreshing your awareness and notice the miracle of being where you are right now, in every moment. To be where you are right now, without judgement about the moment you are in, practice just noticing that you are in it.

Now is the moment I turn on the bath taps.

Now is the moment I stand waiting.

Now is the moment I hang out this sock.

Now is the moment I notice the leaves blowing on the pear tree.

Now is the moment I brush my daughter's hair.

Now is the moment I feel the air filling my lungs.

BEING WHERE YOU ARE
RIGHT NOW: INQUIRY

Practise this noticing just for a moment or two. Although this is the moment you will be writing, you may notice that many more things are occurring in your awareness.

Now is the moment I . . .

Now is the moment I . . .

Now is the moment I . . .

Now is the moment I . . .

What is the effect on you of noticing even these four things?

What is a moment in your day where you typically lose connection to being where you are? What is usually occurring for you in this moment?

Consider how you might practise **being where you are right now** in your day.

What will assist you to remember this practice?

Carry this practice into your day and note below what happens as a result.

44

PLOD, PLOD, PLOD. IS AN ORDINARY LIFE ENOUGH?

*How ordinary this moment can
be, and how extra-ordinary!
We have to keep waking up to
the moment, to the miracle of
our simply being here at all,
so we don't pass through life
somnambulant.*

SPILT MILK

Today, I set the kids up with a DVD and go to meditate for a few minutes. I could do with some heart-transporting bliss, but I don't go anywhere. It is more like treading water. I am holding myself in the tension of being ready to be "Mum" at any moment. I don't allow myself go under, deeper, or let the current carry me. Flotsam drifts past me. Thoughts ebb and flow. I come back to treading water and attempt to stay afloat on my breath. I wonder how long my meditation will be and if I will be interrupted or if I have the stamina to keep going in this ordinary way. It is tempting to give up, but I keep focused on the breath, and it is fine.

I recall sitting in a meditation intensive having a very ordinary experience of meditation. Other people were recounting blue lights and ecstatic explosions of expanding bliss. No excitement for me, though. I was just plain old sitting there, trying to focus my mind on the breath. My meditation seemed so pedestrian. I asked a teaching monk, "Is it happening at all?" She replied, "Look out for spiritual materialism, wanting to have a rush from this or that experience. Some people need a big signal to wake up to something. Some of us have to plod, plod, plod along. Meditation is just what it is for each of us. Just keep going and trust that it is enough."

Back at home, my ordinary meditation continued, plod, plod, plod. I noticed more joy, not during meditation, but in my daily life. A practical, ordinary kind of joy in my day-to-day living.

So today, I'm just getting through. Plod. Plod. Plod. It is good and fine and okay. We get to bedtime, and no one has lost an eye or a limb. But it's so ordinary. Is it enough to live an ordinary life?

Perceiving the Extra in Your Ordinary

Do you believe that the spiritual path is too lofty and solemn for your ordinary day? Do you think you have to induce or evoke some experience other than the ordinary one you are actually having? Don't underestimate the value of the ordinary moment. Even an ordinary moment is an extraordinary moment full of blessings—those many extraordinary moments adding up to your life.

To live your life fully, you must free yourself from expectations and preconceived ideas about what you should or could be experiencing in any moment. Fear and anxiety can get in the way of your being where you are with what is unfolding in the present. Look to the miracle of this moment. What a gift the ordinary moment is! Receive the gift of an ordinary moment by being present in it, alive to the extras contained within it.

The practice here is perceiving the extra in your ordinary. No matter how ordinary you think this moment is, it is the only one you have. As ordinary as it is, this moment is full of the extraordinary blessings of being: of being a mother, of experiencing your senses, of feeling love, of experiencing safety, of freedom from pain.

I wash your face and marvel that we are here together.

I watch you ride your bike and am amazed by your physical learning.

I notice the steam rising from the rice and give thanks for our food.

Awaken to the extraordinariness of this ordinary moment as you wipe your child's face, as you ask for the fourth time that she put her shoes on. See, realise, and appreciate the extra in your everyday blessed ordinariness. This is your extraordinary ordinary life.

PERCEIVING THE EXTRA IN
YOUR ORDINARY: INQUIRY

Take this ordinary moment and practise perceiving the extra that exists in it.

What is the effect on you of doing this?

When in your day could **perceiving the extra in your ordinary** be beneficial?

Carry this practice into your mothering day. Note here the effect it has on you.

What is coming alive in you about the ordinary moments in your mothering day?

AM I DOING IT RIGHT?

Only you can know your inner journey. Only you are responsible for it.

SPILT MILK

I SHOULD meditate for twenty minutes a day. I SHOULD exercise. I should read to my kids, eat healthy, earn enough to feel competent, keep working and build my independent career, enjoy my kids while I can, go on date nights with my husband, keep my house clean and tidy, not care too much, care a lot, look fabulous but without too much effort, cook with my kids, give them extension and stimulation, let them have space to be, monitor their screen time, chill out about being a good mother. I should meditate.

How? When? Should I sit or walk or repeat a mantra? Which one? Shall I use these five minutes to focus on my breath, to contemplate, to try and meditate? Is this chanting working? Would I better off just cleaning the bath right now? Is there any point if I am just sitting listening for my baby to wake up? Is there any such thing as enlightenment? Will my stress damage my children? Put toothpaste on the shopping list. Shall I get up and do that now?

No, I'll just sit. Is that five minutes yet? Am I doing it right? How does anyone do it? What do other people do? Does anyone else find it this hard? If only I had more time, money, childcare, support, this would be easier. Should I journal this?

What does this mantra really mean? Breathe. I'll just breathe. Is that five minutes yet? I feel disturbed by that comment yesterday. I wish I'd said ". . ."

My mind is wandering. Does this even count? Do I even have a spiritual life if I can't sit for five minutes? Don't look at the clock. That's five minutes! But all I did was listen to my anxious mind. It doesn't feel like progress. Was it even meditation? Is there an easier way? Am I doing it right?

Valuing Your Own Journey

What works for your neighbour, your sister, or your friend is what works for them. What worked for your mother, your mother-in-law, your grandmother, and Mother Teresa is what worked for them. It's YOU we're talking about here.

There is a pathway through whatever you are dealing with, but because it is your own journey, you'll have to customise it to match your own circumstances. It is not better or worse than others; it is simply yours. It has its own value.

The practice here is valuing your own journey. Your path is unique, and a big part of walking it is finding what works for you. You will have to test practices and feel what has impact. You will have to trust your own responses, persevere, reflect, be patient, and value each step of your journey as being part of the whole.

When you are in the thick of things and feeling the challenges of mothering so intensely, hold onto the value of having an inner journey. It won't be clear or straight or ready-mapped, but you can be conscious, learning, growing, valuing that you have an intention.

Having embarked on your path of self-inquiry, there is something you must do: value your journey and what arises; value yourself as you pursue living a life of greater wisdom, joy, and purpose.

The path is yours; what practices light your way? You'll know what practices work because they will lead you to feel easier, lighter, happier, and more content for longer. Only you can know that.

VALUING YOUR OWN
JOURNEY: INQUIRY

What is it like for you being a mother today? How come?

What key teaching, practice, thought, or habit currently inspires you on your journey?

What practices have you been testing, or would you like to test?

What have you been discovering?

How do you and how could you **value your own journey** as a mother?

What questions are you currently holding on your inner journey?

46

IF ONLY I HAD MORE _____, I'D BE HAPPY

Storms are inevitable. The more you strengthen your foundation of joy, the more it will weather the storms.

SPILT MILK

Sometimes I think, *If only I had more _____ , I'd be happy*: more money, more time, more clothes, more sleep, more rooms in my house, more things, more holidays, more friends, more love, more joy . . . I warm up to not having enough.

I sit for meditation. I'm going to focus on appreciating the moments of happiness I DO have in my life. It's not all hard work and effort. There are rewards in the moments of joy in amongst it all.

I recall my daughter this morning singing one of her "swing songs" on the wooden swing under the pear tree, head on the side, her little voice floating dreamily among stream-of-consciousness lyrics featuring unicorns and dinosaurs: "I went down to the seaaaa, I made footsteps on the saaaand, I looked out at the seaaaa. Dinosaurs are never gonna be seen. Grrrr! . . ."

I see her freedom, safety, joy. It is a wonderful thing. It gives me great joy to see her in it and to provide safety and love for her. I feel the joy again as I recall it. What a good feeling it is. I love this appreciation of joy. My heart swells. The feeling of joy increases. I love this feeling of joy! It grows so easily! I must do this more!

The more I focus on joy, the more beads of joy I can string on my life more often! It is infectious; I enjoy the carpet I am sitting on, the sound of the birds outside, the joy of breathing in.

It spills over past my meditation time. I am smiling as I prepare our lunch; look at this food! How lucky are we?! My life is very joyous. I want to treasure each moment.

I warm up to abundance. I feel so happy with what I have. I want to live in this awareness more.

Strengthening Joy

Motherhood doesn't have to be all hard work and suffering. Your inner journey doesn't have to focus on your faults and flaws, your wants and failings. Imagine being able to short-cut your struggle and just jump right into your bliss! Well, you can!

The antidote to suffering can be in the simple act of appreciating a cup of tea or a cuddle. Appreciating the tea brings you into the moment where your stories, concerns, and expectations about the past or future can cease. In this present moment, you can become free from the story of suffering. Now you are free to en-joy the tea, to en-joy this cuddle, to en-joy watching your ten-year-old's trampoline flip. You can be joyous while mopping the floor, grocery shopping, washing porridge out of your hair, while sitting, standing, walking, frying onions.

The practice here is strengthening joy. Know it, and grow it. Start with the joy you already have. When you experience a moment of joy in your day, no matter how small, even if it is just a glimpse, hold onto it, focus on it, give it your attention, and let yourself have it fully. Feel the joy and welcome it. That joy is yours. You can keep it. Breathe yourself into it, let it expand, give it your full and nourishing attention. Enjoy it out loud, share it with the world, tell your child, "I am happy! Frying onions in butter smells good!" Own it, strengthen it, have it as many times a day as you want!

So many moments in the day go overlooked, negated, and under-appreciated. When you choose to be joyous, you can even en-joy the things you were telling yourself created your suffering!

STRENGTHENING JOY:
INQUIRY

Recall five of the most joyous moments or times in your life.

List the qualities of each of these moments.

What patterns or themes do you notice to your joy?

Reflect on the core qualities that give you joy. Where do you experience these currently?

Practise **strengthening joy** twice today. Catch a moment of joy, no matter how small. Focus on it, notice what it feels like, where you feel it, and give it your full attention. Describe what happens.

What is one way you could practise **strengthening joy** in the coming week?

47

SURVIVING OR THRIVING?

Gratitude is an antidote to the dark, to judgement, negativity, and despair. Gratitude turns your attention to the light.

SPILT MILK

The morning feels difficult. I am tired. I don't feel resilient. I have to get to Playcentre on time where I'm on duty today. I'm not feeling flowing or on top of things. I'm surviving. I blame myself: *Everyone else seems to manage.* Wherever I turn, mishaps add to a sense of rising pressure. A friend calls; we're both in our early second-child years. "How are you going today?" she asks. We have agreed to share our experience and tell each other the whole truth.

"Well," I say, "my house is a shambles, there's a pool of porridge being tracked onto the carpet, I was up most of the night with a crying baby, my eyes are twitching with tiredness, I'm still in my pyjamas, my fairy unicorn just shut her finger in the drawer so we're about to ice it. Right now she's getting out ice cubes . . . peas . . . ice cream . . . and I have to be at Playcentre in twenty minutes." It feels good to share the reality of our experiences, cacophonic or calm, without fear of judgement. We laugh aloud at the comic farce inherent in our days.

Then, to lift it out of complaint into celebration, we add "BUT HEY . . ." and follow with everything we are grateful for: "At least I don't live in a war zone, no one's lost an eye or a limb today, we're all essentially healthy, we live in a beautiful country, there's a supermarket at the end of the road, excellent national health care service if we need it, we have a roof over our heads, hot running water, food in the cupboard, I have a wonderful husband and a good friend." We have a field day with this last part, naming our many blessings from the grand to the miniscule: "I have two matching socks!" By the end, we are appreciating our great good fortune, laughing at the humour of our blessed predicaments.

I feel lighter, more resilient, accepting, celebratory, and grateful for all I have.

Gratitude

The practice and the result is gratitude. When you identify the things you are grateful for, you recognise the good fortune at the core of your life. It is easy to get caught up in things not being perfect enough, to focus on what is wrong, not meeting expectation, or to see things as holding you back. Use gratitude to locate the solid foundation of your well-being.

Gratitude is transformational, turning challenges into opportunities for learning, obstacles into self-knowledge and wisdom. The practice of gratitude turns your awareness to the miracle of your being alive, toward the abundance, light, and joy in any moment.

Your child is home sick and disrupts your working day? *I am grateful for the flexibility I have to take the day to care for my child.* Over doing laundry and making beds? *I am grateful for dry sheets to sleep in.* Tired of cooking? *I am grateful for the food in my fridge.* Notice yourself rushing distractedly through the shower? *I am grateful for hot running water.* Kids raucous in the car? *I am grateful that even though it is very noisy in the car at this moment, it is happy noise!* Twelve-year-old turns into an aggressive toothpaste-spitting tyrant at bedtime? *I am grateful that I have a mind that will enable a considered response to this unpleasant behaviour.*

With this approach, motherhood fuels your progress on the spiritual path. Simply identifying what you are grateful for will connect you with all that is supporting you in your journey. Gratitude brings you closer to inner peace, to living from a place of patience, forgiveness, understanding, acceptance, and joy.

GRATITUDE: INQUIRY

Make a list of things you are grateful for in your life.

Write down an experience you are grateful for from your day and why.

Recall a challenging moment from your day and see what you can be grateful for in this moment.

What is the effect on you of practising gratitude?

Practise gratitude throughout your day with as many things as you can. Have fun with it. At the end of the day, add three new things you are grateful for here.

Practise this for twenty-one days using the chart at the back of the book. Add three new things to your list every day.

48

I'LL MEDITATE—
AFTER I'VE DONE
EVERYTHING
ELSE

*You will never get everything
done. NOW is the only time
for your love and joy. Making
space for it is the process and
the goal, the transport and
the destination.*

SPILT MILK

My five-year-old has just started school, so she is away now in the days, and my twenty-one-month-old has a day sleep, so when I put her down at around eleven thirty a.m., there is suddenly a GAP!

Time to myself is awash with so much potential that when I realise I have a moment, I panic and go into hyperdrive. I forgo the opportunity I've been longing for to enjoy the space, to meditate, to be still, and fill it instead with work and domestic chores. They're never ending and suck up an hour before I know it. I have to get a grip on this.

I review my endless mental list of Things to Do. "Meditate" is somewhere near the bottom, below "Sort Office," "Clean Bathroom," and "Do Breakfast Dishes."

Today, I'm going to try to suspend the call to do other jobs. Today, I am going to reshuffle that list! Meditation is a priority. When I put baby to sleep at eleven a.m., it will be my time to meditate. THAT is my moment!

I sit. I read something to focus me, then meditate, then journal as time allows. I manage fifteen minutes' meditation. The next day, seven minutes. The next, thirty minutes. The amount of time is not my focus. It is to prioritise making the time and to just do it.

Just doing it makes such a huge difference. Later in my day when I feel overwhelmed or anxious, or when things are chaotic, I focus on my breath. As soon as I turn inward, I am reminded of the lake of stillness I have reconnected to in meditation. I can feel that it is always there, beneath everything. When things are frantic on the surface of my day, I recall the depth of my being and am reassured and steadied just by remembering that it exists.

Making Space by Taking Space

A re you rushing all day to "get it done"? Do you have a sense of too much to do and not enough time, let alone time to meditate? With this approach, you may get lots done, get some of it done, or forever run behind your perpetual to-do list. Then, under the weight and speed of expectations, an overstuffed schedule, never-ending responsibilities, and the many things you are, could, or should be doing in this one moment, you hit a wobble, your hyperdrive function fails, the wheels fall off, and . . . spilt milk.

Trying to get everything done in order to make space in your life is an impossibility, because there will be always be more to do. Here is the truth: there will not be space unless you make it.

The practice here is making space by taking space. Only by taking space for meditation will you make the space it creates. If you want to recharge your batteries, create inner spaciousness, nourish your love and appreciation, and live your moments, minutes, and days of motherhood with a greater sense of joy and ease, then don't finish with meditation—start with it. Rather than thinking, *I'll meditate when I have space*, turn that thought around to *I'll meditate to create space*. Rather than meditating "after everything else," meditate in order to create the state in which you will do all of those other things.

Put "Meditating To Create Inner Spaciousness" on your basics list, like you do "Shopping For Groceries To Eat" and "Reading To My Child For Literacy." If meditation feels like "Yet Another Thing To Do", use it as a break from the list. Take the space to make the space you yearn for, no matter if it is one minute or forty.

MAKING SPACE BY TAKING SPACE: INQUIRY

What is your relationship to meditation?

What benefits do you experience when you meditate?

What gets in the way of you meditating?

What new thoughts and actions could assist you meditating?

When and how could you practise **making space by taking space** in your mothering day today?

Try it and note here how you go.

49

THE
COMPLAINTS
DEPARTMENT

*When we say we want to be happy,
what do we mean? What expectations
do we have of happiness? Do we make
happiness welcome? Do we create
good conditions for happiness? Or
do we expect it will arrive without
invitation, move in, sort out our
lives, take charge, and do everything
for us 24/7, regardless of how
we behave?*

SPILT MILK

Sometimes, I hear my daughter complaining: "The day is too hot. The shoes are too small. The lesson is boring. The hairbrush isn't where it should be . . ." and I think, *Wow, she really has a negative story going there.*

And then I catch myself saying, "The wind is too strong. The dishes aren't done. Now I have to do the washing. I haven't got enough time. They took my parking space. I didn't get enough sleep. Who left that door banging? . . ." Oops.

I'm trying to catch myself in these moments and change my negative feelings into appreciation. But I miss the moment time and time again because I feel so justified in my suffering. *Someone else left that door open to bang and it's annoying me and it's their fault, and I wish they'd just come and close it now and then my life would be better . . .* Really, this does go on, little things ruining my life moment by moment. I know it's not the door or the other person doing it to me. It's me doing it to myself. Complaint is like rust, corroding my joy and peace.

I can choose to be victim to a banging door and an imagined careless person, or I can go and latch the door or choose to not have it bother me. It sounds so obvious, but I have to wrangle my mind and that old victim story!

"The Complaints Department is closing in two minutes, people!" my husband announces. "You have two minutes in which to register all complaints, and then the Complaints Department is shut!" We jump in delightedly with a litany of complaints. It is hilarious and ridiculous and revealing and liberating. The Complaints Department shuts, and we laugh at ourselves and turn toward our happiness.

Choosing Happiness Now

R eady for some shocking news? We can choose to be happy. Reports from the bedsides of the dying is that they realise they could have chosen to be happy with what they had.

What are we waiting for? Let's start now!

The path of yoga promotes freedom from dependency on material wealth and focuses on pursuit of spiritual wealth. It doesn't necessarily preclude material wealth, but having lots of things is not a prerequisite for happiness nor a safeguard against sadness or despair. We cannot be made happy by having a big house, and we can be happy in a tent. Joy and happiness are less about what we have and more about our approach, expectations, and beliefs. Motherhood is a great mirror and a great place to practise choosing happiness over complaint, disappointment, inflexibility, and the multitude of sufferings we inflict upon ourselves.

The practice here is choosing happiness now. If happiness is the cessation of suffering, then you have a choice. You can wait until the world is "perfect" according to your criteria and *then*, when there is no suffering, you can finally be happy. Or you can cease your suffering in this moment by choosing to be happy.

If you ask, "What is the cause of my suffering in this moment?" you may find that the suffering is caused by the idea that things should be a particular way. When the world doesn't match your picture, you might get annoyed at the world, as if the world should comply. If your suffering is caused by disappointed expectations, you have a choice to stop your suffering right now, adjust to reality, and choose to be happy. It is not about simply choosing a positive view; it is about accessing, sustaining, and experiencing your birthright happiness in the life you have now.

CHOOSING HAPPINESS NOW:
INQUIRY

List any complaints you have in your mothering day today.

Choose one complaint from your list. What is the underlying expectation in your complaint?

Restate this situation in a way that frees you to sustain and experience your happiness.

What is the effect on you of writing this?

Take another complaint and do the same:

- write out the complaint
- write out the underlying expectation
- write a new view of this situation that sustains your connection to your happiness

Practise **choosing happiness now** over complaint with something small in your day. Note down what you did and the effect.

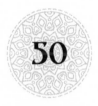

50

STRUGGLING WITH BEING WHERE I AM

No lofty peak is climbed in one stride or without effort. The journey is made by putting one foot in front of the other, step by step.

SPILT MILK

So much of my everyday life as a mother at the moment is step by step. I want to be at ease with the moment-to-moment nature of mothering, but moment to moment, it's such an effort right now.

I feel the compulsory HAVE TO-ness of it. I have to put my own wants on hold and attend to the needs and wants of my children. I have to live the minutiae of the moments, as big and small as they are. I have to be here, present with my children, hand washing, nose blowing, inspecting an ant trail. It is my job; I chose it.

But I don't know how to live MY life for me and at the same time be a mother harnessed to nurturing the lives of others.

I know the journey is in my daily moment-to-moment living and how I am in it. But right now, my life feels like slow drudgery, like I am walking on the spot. It is hard to feel any overall progress. I feel that life is passing me by while I pick up toys or mash pumpkin. I'm on automatic pilot while I herd kids into the bath and read the same book for the 600th time. There is a film of numb frustration between me and my children. My will is flat. My joy is inert.

I'm trying to be steady in the moment so that I am present in my life and with my children. I don't want to miss this time wishing I was somewhere else. I don't want to waste precious time self-absorbed in a struggle with being where I am.

I want to see the step-by-step nature of my day as allowing me to slow down and focus on what is important in each moment. But I am struggling to feel the value of this slow, gluey fatigue in my journey.

Ease with the Moment to Moment

Motherhood is not easy. Days looking after children can feel extremely repetitive, boring, and slow. Mothering demands tolerance, patience, endurance, fortitude, and selfless service. This is even more so in the situation where childcare falls intensely on one person. Your own desires may feel postponed, your individual progress forfeited for others.

Motherhood is a big climb and does require sacrifice and commitment. There will be troughs and peaks, moments of great joy and of great despondency. Maintaining connection to your bigger journey is important.

How do you reap value and opportunity from the grind? What lofty peak are you aiming for as you put one foot in front of the other and trudge uphill against the gravity of your own resistance? Would greater ease with how things are assist you on your journey? Is ease your goal, in fact? If so, here is opportunity.

The practice here is ease with the moment to moment. By its nature, the journey will at times be challenging. Can you be easy with how things are in this moment? You may not want it to be boring or frustrating, and it is easy to appreciate moments that are fun and uplifting, sure, but it is how it is! Don't fight it; embrace it. Use each moment to practise ease: *I am practising ease with this moment of tedium. I am practising ease with this moment of frustration. I am practising ease with this moment of exhaustion. I am practising ease with this moment being other than I want it to be.* The alchemy of adding "ease" to the sentences of your day will transform your larger journey. Try it out!

EASE WITH THE MOMENT TO MOMENT: INQUIRY

What aspect of motherhood are you currently finding challenging? Describe a recent moment that captures this.

What thoughts and feelings were alive in you in that moment?

Describe the moment again, this time adding "ease" to the situation and its challenging aspects.

I am practising ease with this moment of _____.
I am practising ease with this moment of _____.
I am practising ease with this moment of _____.
I am practising ease with this moment of _____.

Practice **ease with the moment to moment** through your day. Say it or write it here and note its effect.

What are you coming to value about the journey of motherhood?

51

GOING IT
ALONE WITH
LONELINESS

*Spirituality doesn't override
biology or psychology; it
complements it.*

SPILT MILK

Today, I feel furious and hurt and frustrated. I feel like I'm holding everybody else's clothes while they go swimming. I've over-accommodated. My needs are coming too far last, too often. And nobody seems to notice or care.

I'm invisible, while I accommodate and adapt and wait for my turn. I've asked nicely. I've even been a bit grumpy. I didn't want to demand; I thought my turn would come at some point if I was reasonable. But I've compromised too far.

I'm deeply hurt and angry. I feel like shouting, "No! I WON'T do that thing to make your life easier. Because it makes mine harder! What about me?! I'm here too! Notice me!" And I feel so ashamed of feeling like this. I should just get over myself. Grow up. But the more I reject the growly monster in the pit of my stomach, the worse I feel. Resentment, jealously, anxiety, fear, and depression surge in my churning gut. I feel alone, desperate, friendless.

What I really want is to be taken seriously. To be valued. Responded to. Cared for. Loved. Held. Appreciated. Engaged with.

How do I get there from this place of despair? I don't want to expose this repellent, weak, hurt, explosive part of me. I should be tougher than this, more competent. I'm a mother, after all!

But I can't just trudge on alone, lobbing stink grenades at loved ones when I can't contain the hurt. Feeling even further away. Sinking.

What would it take for me to reach out? I yearn for connection. But, oh, the pain and risk to break through the membrane of separation and shame and ask for what I need.

Reaching Out to Build Connection

A spiritual life doesn't mean going it alone. A spiritual life doesn't mean being indifferent and emotionless or being above needing others. A spiritual life means embracing what it is to be human and the complexity of our needs. A spiritual life acknowledges the miracle of being, in ourselves and in each other. A spiritual life acknowledges the interconnectedness of things and our need for connection. It asks us to be more, not less, human.

Learning to love and be loved is humanity's spiritual work. Hurt, jealousy, and painful feelings of rejection and exclusion separate us from the love available to us in this world. As a mother, you embody the forces of connection and separation. Motherhood can be intensely lonely, though you may rarely be alone.

The practice here is reaching out to build connection. This means even when you are feeling isolated—especially then. Connecting to others when you feel separate can be a very difficult thing to do. Reaching out when you feel vulnerable may hurt, but it hurts less than not reaching out at all. Why? Because not reaching out moves you further into the dark of your perceived separation, and reaching out moves you toward the light of connection. "I am struggling; I need your help." "I'm trying hard to practise self-responsibility, but I need support." "I feel alone with this; please be with me." "I feel hurt; please hold me." "I feel ashamed of feeling like this. It is hard for me to let you know; please respond."

You are a mother. You are irrevocably connected and inestimably important to your child's life. This is not the time to try and go it alone. Reaching out when you are struggling, asking for help, and trusting the value of building connection is spiritual work, too.

REACHING OUT TO BUILD
CONNECTION: INQUIRY

Describe your current sense of connection. What/who do you feel connected to?

What/who do you feel separate from?

What of these is the most important to you today? Why?

What/who do you want to strengthen connection to, and what could you do to **reach out to build connection**?

Choose one thing you could do to **reach out to build connection** today.

What enables you to **reach out to build connection**?

What gets in the way of you **reaching out to build connection**?

Reach out to build connection today knowing it is a spiritual practice. Note the effect on you. What are you coming to know about yourself?

52

WHAT TO DO WHEN THINGS GO WELL

When a tender shoot of goodness appears, nurture it! Care for it, tend it, clear away the competing weeds, and grow the good things that nourish you.

SPILT MILK

L ife is so good right now. I am loving working at my kitchen table. It is a joyous experience! It is lovely to look out the big window over the valley and watch the weather changing and passing: rain, clouds, wind, stillness, sun, heat, cold, across the trees and hills.

I love my fridge and pantry and being close to it, and the quality of the food I can prepare for myself for lunch and for my family for dinner. We are so blessed! I love having this warm, dry, solid house and the opportunity to write through the days. I appreciate those who support me doing this.

I love my daughters. I love their humour and their deepest selves. I am loving holding and kissing them and being here to care for them. I can feel my own joy in this and can see the benefits that it has for them. I am appreciating learning to let go of my sense of pressure around my children as markers of my own worth. I am loving discovering who my children are as they unfold into the world more and more as themselves, unique and full of potential.

I love my health. I love feeling my strength growing as I put my mind to taking more care of it. I love running, yoga, walking, feeling the capability of my body. I am loving breathing as an antidote to every sense of disease and anxiety.

I love standing still when my daughter rages, knowing I am breaking old patterns of reactivity. I love feeling my solidity and security and knowing that when she has raged and needs to reconnect, she will find me standing just where she left me.

I give thanks for my great good fortune, to be me, learning, here, now.

Growing Goodness

When things are going well, what do you do? Are you so relieved that you leave it at that, taking it for granted that this is how things should be? Or do you stop, celebrate, and appreciate your great good fortune? "Appreciation" means to grow the value of something. You can grow goodness simply by appreciating it.

This is the last practice in *Spilt Milk Yoga*: growing goodness. It is important to acknowledge all that is good in your life.

If you feel resistant to this practice, ask yourself if there is anything you may lose by being appreciative and joyous. Sometimes it is possible that another person may be so invested in you as a collaborator in their misery, that you feel you are betraying them if your life improves or if you are happy. Do you hold back from your own happiness to avoid the anger and envy of others?

Appreciating the goodness of your own unique life helps break habits of comparison and competition and grows a deeper sense of fulfilment and abundance.

It is a worthy piece of work to focus on what is good, no matter how small, to express your gratitude, to give thanks, to notice your joy, to acknowledge, celebrate, and appreciate the richness of your life.

By taking a few minutes in your day to appreciate what is going well, you will live its benefits twice. In addition, the act of appreciation trains your mind to look for the goodness around you.

When things are going well, this is a joyous and uplifting practice. When things are challenging, it is invaluable both to practise and to have already practised.

GROWING GOODNESS:
INQUIRY

Write yourself a letter appreciating all the things that are good in your life.

Read it through. Note the effect it has on you.

*A king once asked his wise
counsellors to give him
something that would remind
him of sadness in joyous times
and of joy in sad times. After
much deliberation, they made
him a ring inscribed with the
words THIS TOO SHALL PASS.*

Afterword

Observing my internal gymnastics and external contortions during the toddler years, my sister told me "It gets easier," and it does. It was encouraging to hear, though it was hard to grasp and apply word of that easier future in any practical way except as a rumour that the intensity would pass. In the overwhelming immediacy of my NOW, I still grappled with being where I was. I wondered how to be in it, with myself, with my children, in the moment to moment of my life, without resisting or wishing it away. I fought to love the preciousness of my NOW.

Now my children are twelve and sixteen, and it's a different world of days. I am not required to meet the same hands-on demands and needs I once did. I sleep in my bed, and they in theirs; they make their lunches, dress themselves, read to themselves, get themselves out the door to school, even make the occasional meal! So, yes, that sort of thing gets easier. Incrementally, my job description as "Mother" has changed. Now I face different concerns and topics to mother through the inevitable joy and sadness, and plenty of old familiar ones visit, too. Toddlers or teenagers, this is just as precious a time to appreciate and experience. This too shall pass.

I know that the quality of my relationship with my children is built on the foundation of hours of cuddles, struggles, frustrations, reconciliations, laughs, and discoveries we have journeyed through together. Mothering still forces me to my edges, and I meet myself there as a determined and loving being, committed to learning and living consciously through all of the spilt milk. I now rank my commitment to mothering to the best of my abilities up there as the greatest achievement of my life.

HABIT-BUILDING CHARTS

HOW TO USE THE CHARTS

1. Select one practice at a time.
2. Make a friendly and manageable goal for yourself.
3. Date your start and begin your twenty-one days of habit-building.

Note: You are learning to habit-build as well as develop this practice. Every day of practice adds up, so don't worry if you miss a day, just start at Day 1 again. By the time you reach twenty-one days, you'll be well on your way!

For the next 21 days, I am practising . . .

Practice	Start Date	1	2	3	4	5	6	7	8	9	10	11	12	13	14	15	16	17	18	19	20	21

For the next 21 days, I am practising . . .

Practice	Start Date	1	2	3	4	5	6	7	8	9	10	11	12	13	14	15	16	17	18	19	20	21

For the next 21 days, I am practising . . .

Practice	Start Date	1	2	3	4	5	6	7	8	9	10	11	12	13	14	15	16	17	18	19	20	21

For the next 21 days, I am practising . . .

Practice	Start Date	1	2	3	4	5	6	7	8	9	10	11	12	13	14	15	16	17	18	19	20	21

For the next 21 days, I am practising . . .

Practice	Start Date	1	2	3	4	5	6	7	8	9	10	11	12	13	14	15	16	17	18	19	20	21

For the next 21 days, I am practising . . .

Practice	Start Date	1	2	3	4	5	6	7	8	9	10	11	12	13	14	15	16	17	18	19	20	21

Acknowledgements

First and foremost, I want to thank my mum, Patricia Monro: thanks for having me. Thanks for always being there, with mind and heart, through every piece of thick and thin we encountered together as mother and daughter, and that we strove, and continue striving, to navigate and embrace. Because of you, I have rarely felt alone.

Thank you to my father, David Monro, for teaching me that love always wins if we keep going, and for daring to take your feisty fifteen-year-old to a Parent and Child Relationships Psychodrama Training weekend. To my sisters, Toni and Briar Monro, thanks for being "Aunty Mum" to my girls and for sharing the whole complex journey, all of it. From playing mums to being mums, we have voyaged the joys, sorrows, conflicts, repairs, and adventures of a life together, with the depth of humour, vulnerability, and love that only sisters can know.

My most profound appreciation to Christian Penny for your commitment to and your belief in my work and the value of this book. You are a wonderful husband, lover, friend, and parenting partner; a wise, playful, and loving father to our girls; my steadfast and insightful supporter at every step; and an inspiring collaborator in every aspect of love and life. You are so truly my other half.

Wholehearted recognition must go to my best-beloved daughters, Ava and Huia Monro, magnificent souls and catalysts of this book. Thank you for the daily life lessons, for all the laughter, cuddles, tears, and learning, and for the richness of opportunities I've had as a mother to stretch my love beyond my previous limits. It is a wondrous satisfaction to witness you growing, unfolding, and carving your own paths. I treasure being your mother, experiencing our special blend of connection, and providing open arms for you to return to as you are, no matter what.

My special thanks to friends near and far: to Sue Morrison for being such a loving and gritty, all-inner-terrain, fellow traveller, and for getting me out of bed and up the hill in all weathers. To Ngapaki Moetara for putting my draft offers to the test so fully; by articulating the value and impact of *Spilt Milk Yoga* on your mothering journey, you strengthened my purpose. To Jo Randerson for your creative, humanitarian, and brave heart. To Lorraine Rastorfer, Andrea Low, and Marilyn Sutcliffe for your nourishing friendship, and to all friends who dared to share the deeper stories of what it truly takes to live consciously as a mother. Thanks to Kate Clere for being a spark-maker, to Kara-Leah Grant for generously sharing your process, to Tara Pradhan for your constancy, to Chardi Christian, who reached out to me at a crucial moment when I was groping in the dark, to Craig Lee for appreciating the little things, to Mary Lou McCombie for your unswerving commitment to presence, to Mike McCombie for your generosity and enthusiasm for the emergent, and to all those who read and talked along the way and contributed with their own stories, questions, and boosts of encouragement.

Warmest thanks to all the good people at Familius: Michele and Christopher Robbins, Erika Riggs, David Miles, Elena Gonzalez, Brooke Jorden, and Sarah Echard, who took such great care in producing a book we can all be proud of. Thanks to the folks at Exisle, especially Lorraine Steele and Alison Worrad, for your straight-talking enthusiasm.

I am grateful to the Ashton Wylie Charitable Trust for the work you do, and to the 2014 judges: Bob Ross, Mike Alexander, and Mary Egan, who saw a book in an incomplete first-draft manuscript. Thanks to Roger Steele for being an early voice of endorsement.

Heartfelt thanks to Max Clayton, Dale Herron, Bridget Brandon, and all my life teachers, great and small; to everyone who contributed through conversations about what matters most—you have taught and inspired me to stand for and follow what is truly important.

ABOUT THE AUTHOR

CATHRYN MONRO is a professional artist, writer, educator, facilitator, and mother of two. She rates mothering as by far the most challenging, creative, important, and fulfilling of jobs. Cathryn's life, training, and work combine her creative drive with a commitment to meaningful education, self-inquiry, group learning processes, and yoga and meditation practices.

Cathryn holds a BFA and MFA from the Elam School of Fine Arts, University of Auckland, and has a 30+ year career as a professional artist. Following her interest in collaboration and communication processes, Cathryn spent a year training as an actor in Sydney, Australia. It was there, in 1990, that she began her yoga and meditation practice.

On return to New Zealand and alongside her studio practice, Cathryn began a 26+ year teaching career in NZ's premiere tertiary arts institutions and trained for 6 years as a facilitator of active and interactive group learning process. She has worked as group facilitator in a variety of educational settings, including with parents for the Anger Change Trust, with teenagers for youth theatre, and as scriptwriter for 11 years for the charity Books In Homes, promoting a love of reading and book ownership to thousands of disadvantaged schoolchildren throughout New Zealand.

In the year 2000, Cathryn gave birth to her first daughter, and in 2003, to her second. Juggling her career and life as a work-at-home mum, Cathryn continued her studio practice, writing, and facilitation, and spent 6 years in hands-on early childhood education with the parent-led Playcentre organization. Over the last 10 years, Cathryn has worked with students and professionals leading integrative, group-learning, practice-based inquiry processes, drawing on the experiences of group members to deepen learning, build collaborative relationships, and enrich working cultures.

Cathryn lives with her husband of 30 years, Christian Penny, and their two daughters in Wellington, New Zealand.

ABOUT FAMILIUS

VISIT OUR WEBSITE: www.familius.com

JOIN OUR FAMILY: There are lots of ways to connect with us! Subscribe to our newsletters at www.familius.com to receive uplifting daily inspiration, essays from our Pater Familius, a free ebook every month, and the first word on special discounts and Familius news.

GET BULK DISCOUNTS: If you feel a few friends and family might benefit from what you've read, let us know and we'll be happy to provide you with quantity discounts. Simply email us at specialorders@familius.com.

CONNECT:
    www.facebook.com/paterfamilius
    @familiustalk, @paterfamilius1
    www.pinterest.com/familius

FAMILIUS

The most important work you ever do will be within the walls of your own home.